Wild Food School

Cooking with
SEAWEED

101+ Ways

Marcus Harrison

First published in 2015 by Marcus Harrison
Lostwithiel, Cornwall. PL22 0ER

Copyright © 2015, Marcus Harrison

ISBN-13 978-1-326-44734-2

CONTENTS

IMPORTANT

Though it is claimed in survival circles that all seaweeds are edible this should not be regarded as the case when it comes to consuming seaweed as daily food. Some species are known to absorb heavy metals and radionucleotides, while some others generate their own anti-grazing compounds.

The seaweed species used in the recipes contained in this book are the better known ones, with a track record of use as human food. Even then, one or two of the seaweeds mentioned have possible caveats attached to them, so moderate consumption of seaweed as part of a well-balanced diet is perhaps the wisest course.

Readers who wish to forage for their own seaweed are advised to make certain they are harvesting from clean coastal environments with pollutant-free waters.

INTRODUCTION

On October 8th 1697, Thomas Allison, Master of the *Ann* from Yarmouth, set sail from the Russian port of Archangel on what was supposed to be a routine return journey to London on behalf of the Russia Company. The voyage became anything but routine, lasting nearly seven months; the *Ann* being forced to seek refuge in a fjord near the North Cape a few weeks after setting sail. For months the small ship and its crew were battered by brutal storms, snow blizzards, and freezing conditions. Crew members suffered from frostbite and were often so numb with cold they were unable to move, while the *Ann's* log suggests the ship's rats even gnawed into the masts to take refuge from the extreme cold conditions.

At one stage Allison is so concerned the harsh frost "*...might render our iron anchors so brittle*," that he leads an on-shore landing party to secure a wooden anchoring post fashioned from a spare mizen mast. Elsewhere, the log notes that Allison shared his personal honey supply so the crew could have hot sweet drinks. In a story which has echoes of Shackleton's heroic exploits of endurance in the Antarctic two hundred years later the *Ann's* crew foraged for whatever they could find on the shoreline when the storms and snow abated, seaweed included.

On February 6th, 1698, Allison records: "*All our men went ashore; some with guns, and among them they shot a white partridge, which was very good meat; the rest employed themselves in gathering muscles, perriwinkles, and dills. These dills are dark brown weeds, growing and hanging upon the rocks, and to be come at while low water: a sort of sea-plant or herb, common enough in the north of England, but more frequent in Scotland. There, I am told, they are eaten raw; but by boiling they become soft, and look greener, tasting not much unlike a colewort. Our way of dressing them was, first, to boil them in fresh water, which took away the saltness natural to them; and after that boiling them again in our beef broth, they supplied the place of a salad, to eat with our beef. By some Scottish men on board, we were happily instructed in the use of these.*"

Elsewhere, Allison conjures up a memorable scene in the ship's galley: "*When night came on, I could not but observe our people as busy, as they are usually in a cook's shop about the Exchange of London, between the hours of twelve and two: only with this difference, that every man was there both guest and servant. This with a kettle, that a saucepan, and the other a dish or platter; some dressing dills, some scallops, muscles, and perriwinkles, and others boiling sea eggs in broth; and some were brewing of mead; so that at both hearths there was scarce room enough for one to get in between to light a pipe...*"

While it may seem strange to start off a modern seaweed cookery book with a tale from the past, it does demonstrate that knowledge of seaweed use among Britain's population was presumably commonplace in some regions, although such tales somewhat cement in the modern psyche the notion that seaweed is purely 'survival' food. Once you get to know your seaweeds you will most certainly decide they are not mere survival food, but a pleasantly surprising culinary ingredient. The *dills* mentioned by Allison is most certainly dulse, although this tends to be categorized as a red seaweed today and has a brown-red to deep purple coloration.

Today, the seaweed industry is big business, though exact figures on production and value are somewhat elusive as the industry is fragmented worldwide. One thing is certain, and that is the vast majority of output goes nowhere near a dinner plate and is destined, rather, for the neutraceutical, pharmaceutical and processed food industries. There the gelling capabilities of the agars, alginins and carrageenans extracted from seaweed allow manufacturers to control the flow, viscosity, and firmness of the products coming off the production line. A whole layer of scientific study is dedicated to researching the gelling properties of seaweeds and is well beyond the scope of this work, as are statistical data on global seaweed production.

If the reader is interested in the scientific aspects of seaweed then the internet is a good place to start, while the United Nations FAO keeps an eye on the global aquaculture business and from time to time produces publications on the subject. However, the purpose of this book is to bring a little seaweed into your life, specifically into your kitchen and diet, with some of the recipes originating in Wild Food School coastal foraging coursework notes from down the years. As you become more familiar with this unusual ingredient you will discover it is not something alien from Mars but is fun to use and can actually taste quite good when prepared properly. So, welcome to the world of seaweeds, and good luck with your explorations.

ABOUT SOME KEY SEAWEEDS

Although there are hundreds of seaweed species found in northern European temperate coastal areas only a small number are really useful (and safe) for culinary use: dulse, laver, various kelps, dabberlocks, sea lettuce, gutweed and Irish moss. These are the main species featured in the following recipes, and probably also the safest to use since they have a long track record of culinary use. As a general rule the thinner species (laver excepted) take less time to cook, or may be eaten raw, while cooking times need to be extended for the thicker and older seaweeds.

From beyond our own corner of the world we also import culinary seaweed species from the Far East, such as wakame, hijiki, arame, and nori. These are generally available in many Chinese, Japanese and other Asian supermarkets and are certainly worth exploring as kitchen ingredients, not least because someone else has done the foraging and gathering on your behalf. These products are also a relatively inexpensive commodity since they come from farmed sources, and are grown on a huge scale in the Far East.

On the scientific and technical side seaweeds are in a world of their own botanically. For some elusive reason seaweeds do not share the same simple physiological nomenclature as their land-based cousins, despite their plant status. The leaf is called a *frond*, the leaf stem is known as a *stipe*, while the rooting part is referred to as a *holdfast*. For identification purposes botanists divide seaweeds into three broad groupings – brown, red and green. The latter ones are often rather delicate and feathery, while the brown group contains some of the toughest and largest species, and the red species (often purple in colour) grow in deeper water since they survive on less light.

Should you decide to forage for seaweed around our own coasts the notes that follow will provide you with a starting point for where to look for the different types and also their appearance. Do be wary of where you forage seaweed from in terms of water quality, as seaweeds have a knack of absorbing toxins and heavy metals. Also work out when the tides work in your favour, and plan your foraging trips accordingly to avoid getting trapped by an incoming tide and becoming an embarrassing news headline. Wear appropriate footwear too, as you will almost certainly need to clamber over rocks at some stage or other during your forage, and wet, seaweed covered, rocks can be tricky and treacherous.

Dabberlocks / Badderlocks – *Alaria esculenta*

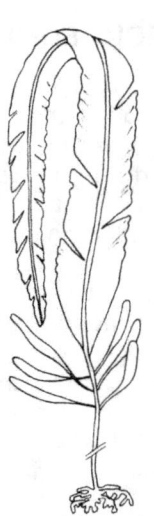

Found growing on rocks at the furthest fringes of the lower shoreline, and in shallow water, dabberlocks is a large brown kelp which grows in cold waters, being unable to survive temperatures above 16°C so is well suited to the waters of northern temperate Europe where it often inhabits rocky, wave-battered, reefs.

Perennial dabberlocks is not as large as some of the other kelps listed here, and at maturity it can reach about 1 metre in length, with the thin frond reaching some 20 cm in width. The rounded stem (stipe) has wing-like branches merging into a distinct, tough, mid-rib that helps provide strength in the inhospitable habitats preferred by dabberlocks.

When young the frond of this seaweed may be eaten raw while material from older species is best cooked.

Tangle / Oarweed – *Laminaria digitata*

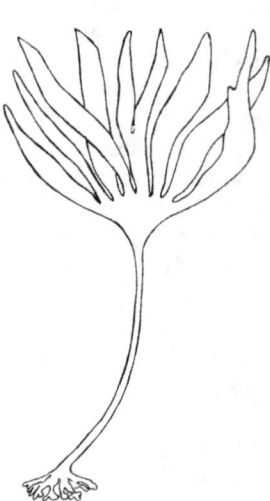

Tangle is one of the larger perennial brown kelp species, reaching lengths of up to two metres sometimes and living for about 3 to 6 years. The stem (stipe) is oval or round in cross-section and is highly flexible, allowing this seaweed to inhabit the rough terrain and battering wave action of the extreme lower shoreline down to about 6 metres.

The broad frond of this species divides into a number of individual finger-like fronds which may be eaten.

Sugar Kelp – *Saccharina latissima*

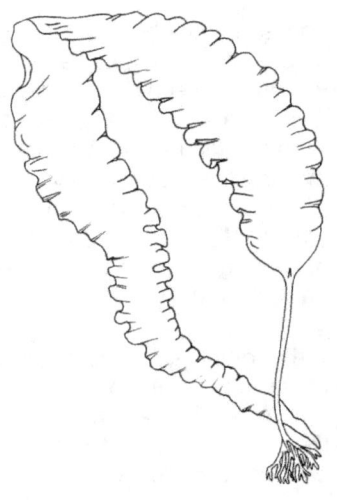

Formerly known as *Laminaria saccharina* this kelp is perhaps one of the easiest seaweeds to identify, having stems (stipes) much shorter than the frond blade itself, as well as a relatively small holdfast. The frond, which may be up to 3 metres long and 20 cm wide, is quite distinctive, having crinkly edges and a long central band somewhat reminiscent of crumpled cloth. Sometimes the central area of the frond is described as having a blistered appearance. Perennial sugar kelp attaches itself to boulders and rocks at the extreme lower shoreline, below low-tide level to depths of about 20 metres. Young specimens are best for food, the main growth dying back each winter.

Sea Spaghetti / Thongweed – *Himanthalia elongata*

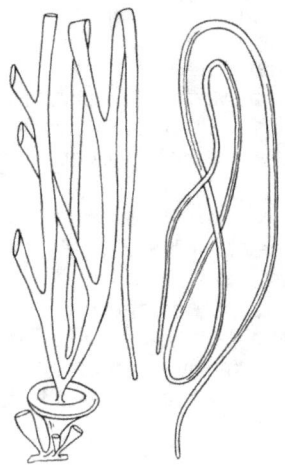

To be perfectly frank I do not rate this edible species very highly, *unless* it is the youngest fronds which are available for use. Older specimens are coarse and, in my view, not really worthy of culinary use – except when deep-fried (see page 81).

Sea spaghetti has long, branched, flattened fronds which may reach 2 metres in length, and are green-brown in colour, although they are a much paler green when very young. Indeed, the early growing holdfasts of this species look like small buttons, from which new fronds sprout. In the early part of the year the rocks upon which sea spaghetti grows are studded with masses of the rather peculiar looking buttons before the fronds sprout.

Laver / **Purple Laver** – *Porphyra* sp.

Sometimes called Purple Laver (*P. umbilicalis*) as opposed to plain Laver, this delicate, thin-leaved, seaweed grows on exposed stones, rocks and timbers at many levels of the shoreline. With fronds growing to about 20 cm long when mature the plant changes colour during the growing season and with age; being purple-violet colour over the winter-spring period but becoming a blackish-olive colour when exposed on rocks later in the year.

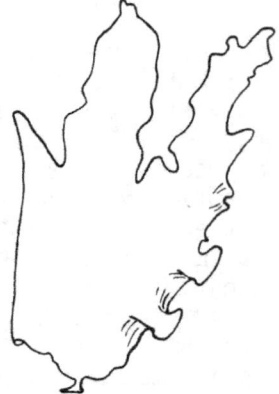

Although laver fronds may feel membranaceous to the touch – being only one cell thick – they are tough and really do need cooking to be made digestible. By comparison the fronds of sea lettuce (*Ulva lactuca*) are two cells thick but are tender enough to be consumed raw.

Many forms of laver exist across the world and in the Far East *P. laciniata* is farmed on a huge scale and is the source of the well-known Japanese culinary seaweed Nori. The square sheets of Japanese nori found in super-markets are produced in a similar process to papermaking; the cleaned *Porphyra* is chopped into small pieces, formed into a slurry, and then poured onto porous matting which allows the water to drain away and then the nori dried. Nori is sold in bundles of sheets called *hoshi-nori*, or as *yaki-nori* when toasted. Nori is often associated with the production of sushi rolls but may also be used soups and as a seasoning, and in Korea is a popular snack accompanying the consumption of beer.

Laver *bread* is made by boiling the fronds in water for a long period until they become a nearly gelatinous green-black mass. This is then formed into blocks for sale, or traditionally (in Wales) mixed with oatmeal, made into patties and fried, or the patties coated in oatmeal and then fried. The dark green purée may also be mixed with olive oil and lemon juice and spread on toast like pâté. Just the sort of thing you might serve up as a canapé at a wild food, or seaweed, dinner party.

Sea Lettuce – *Ulva lactuca*

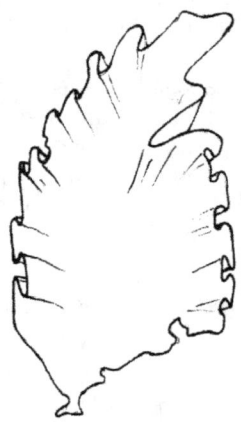

There are a number of *Ulva* varieties around the world but the one most common to us in northern temperate Europe is the annual *U. lactuca*. This species has delicate pale-green fronds (almost like the leaf of a domestic round lettuce) and are translucent enough to see your hand through.

Found growing on rocks and in rock pools from the upper to lower shoreline *Ulva* fronds can reach 40 to 50 cm in length but have no stipe (stem) as such and are attached directly to the rocks. Being such a delicate species sea lettuce tends not to be found (at least in my experience) where the tides and wave actions are strong; unless, that is, a specimen has found a home in a deep rock pool. Sea lettuce can proliferate in the summer months and has a particular liking for fresh-water outlets, especially if they are rich in nutrients (read *effluent* outflows) so care needs to be taken when this is foraged from the coastal areas. Sea lettuce is fine enough to be eaten raw but may also be cooked, and the larger leaves are useful to wrap food in for steaming.

Gutweed – *Enteromorpha* sp.

Gutweed is the name commonly given to one specific member of the *Enteromorpha* species – *E. intestinalis* – though the name appears to be equally applied to other members of the family, *E. linza* and *E. compressa*. The fronds of all these species are tubular and contain pockets of air in varying quantities: *intestinalis* being quite inflated, while *compressa* and *linza* merely have minute bubbles of air trapped in their more flattened tubular fronds. These air bubbles allow *Enteromorpha* to float upright in water – either when the tides are in, or when living in rock pools.

Specimens of *Enteromorpha* are generally found on rocks at the higher tide lines, often looking like a bright green grass covering the rocks and boulders in a shiny mass. They will be found in deeper rock pools of the upper shoreline as well as suitable habitats on the middle and lower shore. Experience shows that *Enteromorpha* is often located in areas where the seawater has reduced salinity levels due to freshwater influence; for example, where there is significant water run-off from fields above rocky shorelines, and in areas of estuarine mud-flats too.

The smallest species of interest, for food, is the thread-like *E. compressa* – having somewhat branched, fine, fronds – while those of *E. linza* are un-branched and rather flattened. *E. intestinalis*, on the other hand, can look quite inflated. In Japan *Enteromorpha* is sold as Aonori along with *Monostroma*, while gutweed is sometimes used crushed or powdered.

Dulse – *Palmaria palmata*

Also referred to scientifically as *Rhodymenia palmetta* dulse was touched upon in the Introduction to this book, and is perhaps one of the best known common seaweeds with a long history as an edible seaweed in temperate Europe and other parts of the world; young fronds being cooked with potatoes, in soups and fish dishes, eaten dried as a snack, smoked, or ground for seasoning.

Brownish-red to purple in colour, perennial dulse grows on rocks from the mid-to-lower shoreline, sometimes to 20 metres depth, being also found attached to the stalks of larger kelp species. The fronds are pretty tough and leathery, flat, and grow on a small stem (stipe) from a small holdfast. They range between 10 to 50 cm in length and 3 to 8 cm wide, and lack a midrib.

Irish Moss / Carragheen – *Chondrus crispus*

Irish Moss, in my view, is not really one of the edible, vegetable-like, seaweeds. Rather, it is the source of a vegetable alternative to gelatine (known as carra-geenan) which is handy for vegetarian diets. That said, the extraction process from the physical seaweed is long-winded and any reader keen to experiment with seaweed gelling agents would be better off heading to a Chinese or Asian shop and buying *agar agar* which is far simpler to work with.

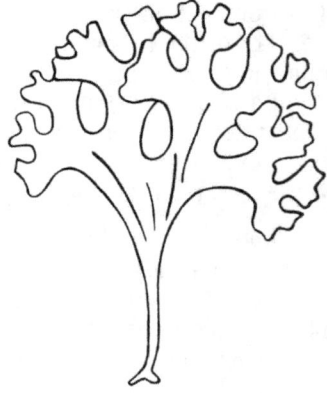

As a starting point for Irish Moss try about 20 to 25g of the dried seaweed to 1 litre of water, boil for 45 to 60 minutes then strain and use the liquid to set a jelly. Precise times and quantities can vary depending on the gelling qualities of the seaweed batch. Before you head off to make a jelly in this way it is worth pointing out there have been some health concerns over the carrageenans in Irish moss. So if that is a concern do some research on the web.

Irish moss is a purple-red perennial species, the fronds growing up to about 15 cm in length and the plant finding a home on the stones and rocks of the lower shoreline, in rock pools and shallow water.

Pepper Dulse – *Laurencia pinnatifida*

Pepper dulse is included here for its potential use as a seasoning rather than as a vegetable food, although it has been eaten in that form in the past when specimens are very young. It can be very coarse and rough and is far better dried and then ground into a spicy seasoning, in my view.

The ten, or so, varieties of seaweed above are those commonly found around Britain's shores and the coastlines of much of northern temperate Europe. However, there are other exciting sources of different seaweeds to be found in Asian supermarkets, some of which are detailed below.

The Far East has a long track record of seaweed consumption and some of the farmed output is exported to distant corners of the world. Japan, Korea, and increasingly China, have large seaweed industries, the produce of which may be used for chemical compounds, at others times as gelling agents for the processed food and pharmaceutical industries, and also for your dinner plate.

If the prospect of expending energy on foraging for your own seaweeds leaves you feeling daunted then purchasing the imported seaweed types below may provide you with a good solution. Some of these may be substituted for the European seaweed species in some instances, and I have indicated where I think this to be the case. These dried imported seaweeds offer good value for money, and if you like to explore new foods then I think you will have a lot of fun. *Wakame*, in particular, is a good starting point to explore these new ingredients. I recently gave two friends, who were rather sceptical at the thought of consuming seaweed, a little wakame to try and they were both really pleasantly surprised. Thinking about it, if you are really reticent about seaweed as a foodstuff, and you live in a city where there is an Asian supermarket, may I suggest investing in a packet of dried *wakame* as a low-cost starting point? If you find that you like the taste of your small investment then you have started on your seaweed journey, but should you hate the taste or texture then you know not to invest further time or money. The famous *nori*, used in sushi, is omitted from the list below since it is essentially a shredded form of laver (often *Porphyra yezoensis* and *tenera*) touched on previously, while dried Far Eastern laver is often available in thin, cake-like, packs.

Kombu – *Laminaria* species.

Kombu is the Japanese name for the dried seaweed derived from a variety of kelp species, the key ones being *L. longissima, japonica, angustata, coriacea,* and *ochotensis*. Like the European kelps, kombu species are generally too thick and robust to digest raw and need extended cooking times – sometimes hours – unless you happen to be working with very young specimens.

Japanese cooks make a soup stock, known as *dashi*, from kombu and dried bonito (tuna) flakes, which finds its way into lots of Japanese dishes. In European Asian supermarkets dried kombu is generally available in both sheet and cut form, and also as 'bows' – slivers of kelp tied in knots.

Wakame – *Undaria pinnatifida*

In its native habitat wakame has physical similarities to dabberlocks (*Alaria esculenta*); having a broad, lance-shaped, frond with a prominent midrib, with the segmented fronds reaching 1 to 3 metres in length. The stem (stipe) of wakame, on the other hand, is smooth while that of *Alaria* is corrugated. Both are classified as brown seaweeds.

The dried commercial form of wakame (granular or short lengths) for domestic kitchen use has an appearance somewhat reminiscent of the black leaves of green tea, but when the pieces are rehydrated in water they just seem to explode in size, becoming green in colour also. Very often I consider a tablespoon of dried wakame as more than enough for a one person serving. To my mind wakame is a good substitute for sea lettuce, being edible both raw and cooked. From what I understand, but have never experienced, the *holdfast* (root) of wakame is sometimes eaten in Japan; dried, cut into slivers, and then eaten with miso.

14

Hijiki / Hiziki – *Hizikia fusiformis*

This is a brown seaweed which looks black once dried for domestic use and, unlike wakame, needs a long boiling or steaming time before it is used, and must obviously be rehydrated first (for about 30 minutes). As with wakame dried hijiki expands enormously when reconstituted with water. The fronds, which reach about 15 cm in length, are string-like rather than flat, and I have used them as a substitute for sea spaghetti in terms of their strand-like visual appearance. However, hijiki can be rather salty, and the black worm-like strands might unnerve your faint-hearted dinner guests unfamiliar with eating seaweed.

One final point about hijiki is that health concerns have been raised in Japan regarding the safety of this seaweed for human consumption, based on hijiki's high absorbtion levels of arsenic. While this has not resulted in an outright ban on consumption the advice is to consume hijiki in moderation (just like any food really). There is bound to be plenty of information available on the web, so if you are concerned then do some personal research. It is a good reminder, too, that seaweed should be eaten sensibly.

Arame – *Eisenia bicyclis*

Arame is categorized as a brown algae and is one of the milder tasting seaweeds, having a very mild sweetness in taste. These qualities make arame suitable for many dishes while also making it a good starting point for those just starting their explorations into the world of edible seaweeds. Like the other Asian seaweeds here arame is supplied in dried form, with the dark brown to black strands of the fronds rehydrated in water for 5 to 10 minutes, and then used in salads and soups. A native seaweed of Japan, where it typically grows on reefs, arame's delicate fronds may reach about 60 to 70 cm in length.

Kanten / Agar Agar

Kanten is not a seaweed but a seaweed-derived gelling product, available in sheet, shredded and powdered forms. More readily known as agar, or agar agar in the west, kanten is tasteless, apparently has zero calories, and provides an alternative option to animal gelatine for use in both savoury and sweet dishes. In my view the process of reconstituting agar in water is far easier than boiling up Irish Moss for hours to extract the gel. There's more about the culinary use of agar / kanten on page 122.

SEAWEED PREPARATION and THE RECIPES

The recipes which follow are designed for use with the European sea-weed species listed towards the front of this book; being tried and tested over time and relatively safe, while some of the Asian species may be substituted here and there. There are, however, **some important factors to observe when interpreting the recipes** as they are written. Indeed, most are are written with a somewhat open, broad, canvas. This is because some readers will be working with freshly foraged seaweed while others may be using shop bought punnets of seaweed, or even seaweed in dried form. For the most part the recipes are for 2-person servings, allowing you to trial them on a manageable small scale before enlarging quantities to feed larger numbers.

In every case – unless a recipe specifies *dry* seaweed – then the assumption is that you are working with a hydrated or rehydrated sea vegetable. Where you are working with freshly gathered seaweed then it is recommended you rinse your produce to remove excess salt before starting your culinary explorations. Shop bought dried seaweed is often cleaned with fresh water before drying so the salt content is already lower. It's just a question of familiarizing yourself with the brand or source.

You also need to become familiar with the properties of individual species – as you are with carrots or potatoes – and how they cook up. What I suggest is that until you become familiar with cooking seaweeds you alter (where possible) the cooking *method* of a recipe and pre-cook the seaweed component and then recombine it with the other ingredients at a later stage in the cooking procedure.

If you are foraging for your own seaweeds then you need to under-stand when individual species are at their toughest or most tender in their annual life-cycle. For example, if I am using foraged kelp I personally never use anything but the youngest fronds for the kitchen. Where older seaweeds are the only resource available then you need to approach them with longer, slower, cooking times. Old seaweed is essentially indigestible.

Regarding salt in the recipes. Although seasoning is mentioned in some of the recipes I more often leave salt *out* of the main cooking procedure and then adjust or add salt afterwards before serving. This is because you cannot always guarantee the saltiness of fresh seaweed even if it has been soaked in fresh water before use. And, in any case, too much salt is probably bad for you. Incidentally, the soy sauce used in the recipes is nearly always the *light* variety, while sunflower oil is mainly specified in preference to olive oil. The logic behind this is that it allows you the opportunity to taste the seaweeds in as clean a tasting form as possible the first time you try a recipe; avoiding the masking flavour of olive oil, particularly the extra virgin kind. Once you have tried the recipe then you have the option of switching to olive oil next time.

Speaking of *bad* things before. When foraging for your own seaweed supplies make sure it comes from an area with no water contamination or pollutants, as some seaweeds absorb toxins and heavy metals. Similarly, I would stick with the tried and tested species mentioned in this book as some seaweeds are known to contain suspect chemicals (*Dilsea carnosa*, for example), and are not recommended for consumption, or certainly long-term consumption. This would also apply to those seaweeds which have ultra-high iodine levels since an excess of iodine is as bad as a lack of it. In many respects I do not regard seaweed as a typical vegetable to be consumed in large quantities, as one would cabbage, potatoes, carrots or other common domestic vegetable.

The other aspect of safety concerns the place you harvest from. Wet, seaweed covered, rocks are treacherous, as are tides. So be careful when foraging for your own seaweed stocks.

Another point certainly worth mentioning is that humble seaweeds, like their land-based counterparts, have annual, biennial and perennial life-cycles depending on the species. So it is important to think *sustainably* when seaweed foraging. Only take *part* of the leaf fronds, particularly in the case of annual seaweeds (like sea lettuce), since the fruiting bodies of seaweeds form on the fronds that you want to eat. By taking the whole frond you have interrupted the reproductive cycle. With some perennial seaweeds, like dulse, new growth will appear from the cut edge of the previous season's leaf. Even with the bigger kelps leave the holdfast (root) and stipe (stem) intact, cutting the fronds you want for the kitchen a few inches above the end of the stipe. This allows new growth to regenerate. And don't be too greedy when you are harvesting. Seaweeds are part of an ecosystem; mostly out of view beneath the waves but still the habitat and food for many other living organisms.

Finally, you will notice in the layout of this work there is lots of white space between the recipes, some of which derive from Wild Food School foraging coursework. This layout is quite deliberate because it is imagined that until you become familiar with the seaweeds listed then you will need to make notes about your culinary adventures, and changes or amendments to the recipes. So regard this book more like a workbook, writing your notes in the extra spaces, and the recipes as starting points.

SOUPS

SEASIDE SOUP

1 small onion, chopped
Butter or oil
1 medium potato, cubed
1 small carrot, diced
½ cup wild greens (optional)
½ cup seaweed
Water
Salt and pepper

A slowly cooked soup can be a good way to make dabberlocks fronds, or sections of young sugar kelp fronds, more easily digested. On the other hand, changes to the cooking time lend this recipe to the tender fronds of sea lettuce – or even commercially available wakame.

If using kelp, shred it small first – around matchstick size. Sea lettuce can be in larger chopped pieces. I suppose you could make this a smooth soup and blitz the final cooked ingredients, but somehow it looks nicer with all the different colours, and provides a medley of textures. Down to you really.

• Fry the onion until softened then add the carrot and potato, and stir-fry until the vegetables begin to take on a little colour.

• Next, add the seaweed (and any other wild veggies) and enough water to cover the ingredients.

• Bring to the boil and cook for a few minutes, then reduce to a simmer, cover, and cook until the potatoes and carrots are done. Serve.

BEAN and SEAWEED SOUP

1 small can canellini beans, drained
1 small shallot, chopped
Oil
1 medium potato, diced small
Garlic purée, to taste (optional)
2-3 cups vegetable stock
¼-½ cup seaweed – sea lettuce, dabberlocks or laver
Pepper

Use tender young laver fronds for this, young dabberlocks with the midrib removed, or any of the more tender edible green seaweeds. Where laver is being used then the cooking time may need extending considerably. The best advice with laver is to pre-cook it until the preferred level of tenderness is achieved, then incorporate it into the recipe.

• Begin by finely shredding the seaweed. Set aside.

• Next, in a heavy-bottomed pan fry the shallot until it starts to soften, then add the diced potato and sweat for about 10 minutes; stirring to prevent the pieces sticking to the pan.

• Then add 2 cups of the stock, a little garlic purée, and the seaweed, and bring to the boil for a couple of minutes.

• Reduce the heat to a simmer and cook for another 10 minutes, adding more stock if required. Serve.

CHICKPEA and SEAWEED SOUP

½ cup young sugar kelp or dabberlocks, chopped
1 small shallot, chopped
Garlic purée, to taste (optional)
1 tsp. root ginger, finely grated
Sunflower oil
1-2 tsp. garam masala
3-4 cups vegetable stock
1-1½ cups cooked chickpeas
Dried laver, finely crushed or minced

• Drop the seaweed pieces into boiling water and cook for 5 minutes, then drain and set aside.

• Fry the shallot in a little oil until it softens, then add the garlic and ginger and cook for another couple of minutes; stirring to prevent burning.

• Add the garam masala, and stir for 30 seconds.

• Add the stock and seaweed, and simmer for 10 minutes.

• Next, add the chickpeas, and cook for 5 minutes, then blend with a hand-blender (to the consistency your prefer – or leave thick and chunky).

• Stir in a teaspoon of crushed laver, leave for a couple of minutes, and garnish with more crushed laver for visual effect then serve.

CARROT and SEAWEED SOUP

Unsalted butter or oil
1 small shallot, chopped
2 large carrots, chopped
1 small potato, chopped
1 pint chicken stock
½ tsp. ginger root, finely grated
½ cup dulse, finely chopped
Double cream (optional)

• Sweat the chopped shallot in a little butter or oil until softened.

• Next, add the carrot, potato and stock. Bring to the boil then reduce the heat to a simmer and stir in the grated ginger.

• Cover the pan and simmer for 15 minutes.

• Then remove from the heat and blitz the soup ingredients with a hand blender.

• Return the pan to the heat and add the chopped dulse and continue to simmer gently for another 5 to 10 minutes.

• Stir in a spoon or two of cream, if using, and serve.

SEA LETTUCE CHOWDER

1 medium potato, peeled and sliced
1 small onion, finely chopped
Water
2 or 3 sea lettuce fronds, washed, shredded or cut into shapes
White fish fillet
Milk, splash
Butter

Depending on how soft you like your sea lettuce consistency combine it with the potato and onion in the first step (softer), or add along with the fish fillet later in the cooking procedure (giving the seaweed a more crunchy texture).

• Place the potato and onion in a pan with about a pint of water and bring to the boil, then reduce the heat and simmer until the potatoes start to soften.

• Add sea lettuce first and then layer the fish fillet over.

• Raise the heat for a minute or two, then reduce, cover the pan and cook until the fish is done.

• Finally, stir in a splash of milk and a small knob of butter, and serve.

CURRIED SEAWEED, POTATO and CLAM CHOWDER

½ cup sugar kelp or dabberlocks
1 small onion, chopped
Sunflower oil
2 medium potatoes, diced small
1 pint fish stock
¼-½ tsp. medium curry powder (or paste)
Pepper
1 small tin of baby clams, drained

• Chop or cut the seaweed into small squares or strips – depending on presentation preferences – having first removed the midrib.

• Fry the onion in a little oil until soft, then remove from the pan and set aside.

• Add the potatoes, seaweed pieces, curry powder and fish stock.

• Bring to the boil for a couple of minutes, cover, then reduce the heat and simmer for 12 to 15 minutes, or until the potatoes are tender. For a little more thickness mash some of the potato with a masher at this point.

• Add the drained baby clams to the pan, and cook for another 2 or 3 minutes until the clams are heated through.

MACKEREL and SEAWEED CHOWDER

1 cup fresh mackerel meat
1 small onion, chopped
¼-½ cup sea lettuce or gutweed, finely chopped
Oil
2-3 tsp. plain flour
2-3 cups skimmed milk, warmed
Dried laver, finely crushed
½ cup canned sweetcorn kernels, drained
Ground paprika or chilli

For this recipe use freshly caught mackerel as it is a wholly different ingredient than the prepared, shrink-wrapped, product bought off a supermarket shelf. On one occasion I also prepared this with ling, which has a somewhat bland flavour and needed chilli levels boosting to compensate.

• Begin by cutting the fish into small pieces.

• Next, sweat the onion in a heavy-bottomed pan until it is soft. Then stir in the seaweed and cook gently for several minutes.

• Sprinkle the flour over the mixture, combine thoroughly, and cook for about a minute.

• Add the warmed skimmed milk a bit at a time; stirring to ensure no lumps form.

• Stir in a sprinkle of the crushed, dried, laver.

• Raise the heat to a gentle simmer then add the mackerel, and cook for 10 minutes.

• Next, add the canned sweetcorn and cook for a further 3 or 4 minutes.

• Season with chilli or paprika to taste, and serve.

SEAWEED-BULGUR BROTH

¼ cup onion, finely chopped
Sunflower oil
Paprika or chilli powder, large pinch
3 or 4 cups vegetable stock
1-2 tbsp. bulgur wheat
¼ cup young dulse and/or sea lettuce, chopped
Salt

• Start by frying the onion until translucent and it begins to brown, then add pinches of spice and cook for another minute or two. Set aside.

• Place the stock in a pan, bring to the boil, then stir in the bulgur and turn down the heat to a simmer.

• Stir in the seaweed and allow to cook through for a further 10 to 15 minutes.

• Add extra seasoning as required, then serve.

FISH BALL and SEAWEED SOUP

1 cup skinless white fish, boned
3 tsp. cornflour
¼-½ garlic clove, minced
¼ red chilli, finely chopped
1 medium egg white
¼-½ cup sea lettuce / gutweed
3-4 cups water
Vegetable stock cube
Pepper
Tofu, spring onion, mushrooms (optional)

When living in London I would buy ready-made fishballs from the super-markets in Chinatown for simplicity, but if you are worried about the ingredients in commercially supplied fishballs then you can always make your own, and there are plenty of recipes available. I prefer to chop the fish by hand as, in my view, using a blender tends to produce a paste too fine texture-wise, but that is a personal choice. Likewise, I would avoid using garlic purée as that also contributes to a soft texture.

Other ingredients you may like to add to the liquid soup base are tofu (small cubes or sliced), spring onion and thinly sliced button mushrooms, although chestnut mushrooms also add a nice taste.

• Begin by mincing the fish very finely, then place in a large bowl with the chilli, garlic, and egg white, and mix thoroughly with a fork.

• Next, sprinkle in the cornflour a little at a time and mix in until a sticky mass forms.

• Take handfuls of the paste and throw or slap it back against the bowl sides repeatedly until it becomes less sticky, and somewhat springy as air is incorporated into the paste. Then cover the bowl with cling film and chill in the refrigerator for 30 minutes.

• Meanwhile, place 3 cups of water in a pan (reserving one cup), and dissolve a stock cube in the water.

• Wash and finely shred the seaweed.

• Once the fish paste is chilled, bring the stock to the boil. If using tofu, spring onion or mushrooms, add these to the pan now. Add a little pepper seasoning (or more chilli, cayenne or paprika for varying degrees of heat).

• Take dessert spoon portions of the fish paste, form into small 1-inch balls, and lower gently into the boiling stock. They are done when they rise to the surface and float, usually about 3 to 4 minutes.

• Add the seaweed and cook for 4 or 5 minutes more, then serve.

SEAWEED, NETTLE and TOFU SOUP

¼-½ cup young sugar kelp, finely shredded
2 handfuls very young nettle leaves
2-3 cups water
1 small shallot, chopped
1-2 tsp. grated ginger root
½ tsp. ground cumin
Sunflower oil
Salt and pepper
2 oz tofu cubes

Young springtime nettle growth should coincide with the young growth of many seaweeds, and also ramsons (*Allium ursinum*), a type of wild garlic that grows in hedgerows and could also be added to the ingredient list.

• Begin by shredding the sugar kelp very finely, place in a pan with 2 cups of water, bring briefly to the boil then simmer for 10 minutes, or until cooked.

• Remove the seaweed from the pan with a slotted spoon, and set aside.

• Boil the nettles in the residual water, adding the third cup of water. Cook for five minutes, then turn off the heat.

• Meanwhile, fry the shallot in a small amount of oil until soft, and then stir in the ground cumin and ginger. Cook for a few minutes, stirring to prevent the spice ingredients scorching.

• Add the fried shallot mixture to the cooked nettles and then blend the contents of the pan with a hand blender. Add extra hot water to achieve the soup consistency preferred, and add seasoning to taste.

• Turn up the heat again, add the shredded kelp, cubed tofu, and cook for a few more minutes to warm through. Serve.

FISH SCRAP CHOWDER with SEAWEED DUMPLINGS

1-2 cups raw fish meat / shellfish
3-4 cups fish, or vegetable stock, hot
1 small shallot, chopped
Sunflower oil
1 tomato, skinned and sliced
1 red pepper, de-seeded and chopped
Garlic purée, to taste
Saffron, small pinch and chopped
Seaweed (optional)

1 egg yolk
1-2 tbsp. milk
½ cup plain flour
½ tsp. baking powder
¼ cup sugar kelp, dabberlocks or sea lettuce
Butter

This recipe is designed to use up all those bits of fish and shellfish which may be left over from another larger fish recipe you have been preparing. Similarly, any fish tails, heads, lobster or crab shells can all be cooked up for 30 minutes to provide the basis for a stock to be used here. Essentially this recipe is about ensuring that nothing from your catch goes to waste. Vary the thickness, or chunkiness, of the end result by increasing the amount of fish or shellfish used. To give the chowder a spicy twist, add a few drops of Tabasco sauce – the red variety for lots of heat, or the green type for a more mellow heat.

Seaweed dumplings are something that do not really go with much else other than a fish soup, chowder, or fish stew. Use one of the more tender seaweed varieties, or pre-cook the more substantial ones then incorporate into the recipe. In the case of mild tasting sea lettuce the seaweed is used for its visual effect in the dumplings rather than taste. For something more robust replace sea lettuce with dulse. Another alternative is to dispense with the dumplings and add seaweed as a chowder ingredient in its own right.

• Begin by stripping the fish meat from bones, and preparing fish stock from leftovers – if you are doing this.

• Fry the chopped shallot in a little oil until softened and transparent, then stir in the tomato, red pepper, garlic purée and saffron and cook for a few minutes more.

- Add the hot stock, bring to the boil, then simmer for 10 to 15 minutes.

- Next, add the fish ingredients and a little seasoning, and continue to simmer for 15 minutes.

- After adding the fish ingredients start to prepare the dumplings (the second batch of ingredients) by finely shredding the seaweed. Set aside.

- Next, sift the flour and baking powder into a bowl, along with a pinch of salt.

- Beat the egg yolk with the milk and set aside.

- Warm a knob of butter then rub it into the flour mixture until this has the appearance of a crumble pastry mixture.

- Add the chopped seaweed and mix in with a fork.

- Give the egg-milk mixture a stir then add to the combined flour-seaweed ingredients, and mix through with a fork until a dough forms.

- Drop spoonfuls of the dough into boiling salted water, cover the pan, and cook for 10 to 15 minutes, or until done (the dumplings will float).

- Serve the dumplings with the chowder.

DRIED LAVER SOUP

1 pint vegetable stock
1 small spring onion
1 small shallot
1-2 tbsp. dried laver, finely crumbled

Although laver is very thin, it is a tough seaweed which requires and extended cooking time. For it to be used more like a vegetable it is best to crumble or powder the dried seaweed which makes it more digestible.

• Slice the spring onion into narrow rings, and similarly the shallot.

• Place the stock in a pan and bring to the boil.

• Add the spring onion (reserving 1 tsp. of pieces), shallot and laver to the pan. Allow to boil for a couple of minutes, then reduce to a simmer, cover, and cook for 20 to 30 minutes.

• Serve with the reserved spring onion pieces sprinkled over.

SALADS

SPICY DULSE SALAD

½-1 cup young dulse, roughly chopped
Dried chilli flakes, small pinch
1 tsp. rice wine vinegar
½ tsp. light soy sauce
1 tsp. sesame oil
Salt, as required
1 tsp. clear honey
White sesame seeds

Use the very youngest dulse fronds you can find for this recipe. Raw sea lettuce can be used as an alternative, as could commercially produced wakame.

• Wash the dulse to remove excess salt, pat dry on kitchen paper, and place in a bowl.

• Mix all the seasoning ingredients in a small dish, drizzle this over the dulse, toss, and serve as a side salad or accompaniment to a fish dish.

DULSE SALAD

Dried dulse
Apple, cored, quartered and sliced
Cucumber, peeled, diced
Walnuts, chopped
Cider vinegar
Lemon juice
Olive oil

This salad recipe is very open ended, essentially allowing you to use whatever proportions of the main ingredients you like, though the walnuts generally want to be in a smaller quantity.

• Begin by soaking the dried dulse in water for about 10 to 20 minutes to soften, then drain, shred and place in a bowl.

• Add the cucumber, apple, and chopped walnuts and mix thoroughly.

• Finally, make a dressing of 1 part each of lemon juice, cider vinegar and oil, drizzle over the ingredients in the bowl and toss.

DLT

Ripe tomatoes, chopped
Iceberg lettuce, shredded
Dried dulse, shredded
Mayonnaise
Dijon mustard (optional)
Lemon juice
Chorizo, sliced (optional)

DLT meets BLT. Yes, it's time for dulse as a stand-in for bacon. This is a short salad recipe which I have used for years as a way of introducing foraging novices to the alien concept (at least in their eyes) of eating sea-weed as food.

The basic concept here is to use the saltiness of dried dulse as a bacon alternative, although there was no intention of making this a vegetarian recipe. For meat eaters the addition of some fried chorizo slices provides a spicy accent for a change.

Readers absolutely wedded to having their traditional BLT between two pieces of bread or toast can put their DLT in a taco wrap, or even steamed rice paper wraps like a Chinese spring roll.

• De-seed the tomatoes, slice neatly into small pieces and place in a mixing bowl.

• Add the shredded lettuce to the bowl, and the dulse too.

• If using the chorizo option, slice the sausage thinly then lightly fry to release the fat, then remove from the pan with a slotted spoon and add to the mixing bowl. [Alternatively the chorizo pieces may be used as a garnish.] Mix the ingredients to distribute them evenly.

• In a small dish place a couple of tablespoons of mayonnaise, then add a little lemon juice to thin it, and a small quantity of mustard (optional). Mix, drizzle over the salad mixture, toss and then serve.

DULSE-ORANGE SALAD

1 small / medium orange, juiced
½-1 cup dried dulse
1 tbsp. toasted sesame oil
Tabasco sauce, to taste
Toasted sesame seeds

Do not leave the dulse soaking too long in the OJ as it tends to become soggy.

- Place the orange juice in a bowl.

- Add the dulse – torn into manageable pieces – and push beneath the orange juice.

- Add in the sesame oil and a little Tabasco to add a spicy touch, and mix everything through with a fork.

- Allow the dulse to soak in the dressing for around 5 to 10 minutes, then serve with some toasted sesame seeds sprinkled over.

DULSE and CORN SALAD

2 cups cooked sweetcorn
¼ cup dried dulse, shredded
¼ cup sea lettuce, chopped (optional)
Garlic purée (optional)
2-3 tsp. sunflower oil
1-2 tsp. lemon juice

This is an accompaniment rather than a main dish, and uses dried dulse to provide both saltiness and flavour, while the optional sea lettuce may be replaced by wakame. The presence here of garlic – to personal taste – is very definitely an individual matter, so the suggestion is to try this recipe without garlic first time round. Canned sweetcorn is also ideal for this recipe.

• Place the sweetcorn in a bowl.

• Add the seaweed ingredients and fold through with a fork.

• In a small dish make a dressing with the lemon juice and oil (adding garlic to taste, if using).

• Drizzle the dressing over the ingredients in the bowl, mix through, and serve.

SEAWEED, CABBAGE and APPLE SALAD

½ cup white cabbage, shredded
¼ cup dulse, shredded
½ orange, juiced
2-3 tsp. apple cider vinegar
1 apple

Use a firm and good-tasting eating apple species for this. Orange Pippin, Golden Delicious, Braemar or for example.

• Place the cabbage and dulse in a bowl, and mix.

• In a separate small bowl mix the orange juice and cider vinegar.

• Thinly slice the apple, dropping the pieces into the orange-cider mixture, and from time to time fork the pieces over.

• Add the apple mixture to the cabbage and dulse, distribute the ingredients thoroughly with a fork and serve.

DULSE TARTARE

Dried dulse, finely chopped
White wine vinegar
1 tsp. spring onion (white part), finely chopped
2 tbsp. mayonnaise
½ tsp. Dijon mustard

For simplicity, bought mayonnaise is used for this recipe, but equally you could make your own with egg yolks and olive oil. Serve with fried fish, or other fish dishes.

• Place the finely chopped dulse in a small dish and add just enough vinegar to cover. Allow the seaweed to rehydrate for about 10 minutes, then drain off any excess vinegar.

• Add the spring onion to the dish and mix in.

• Then stir the mayonnaise and mustard into the mixture and distribute evenly.

DULSE MARMALADE

1 small red onion (or red shallot), sliced
Olive oil
1-2 tbsp. fine brown sugar
¼-½ cup dulse, chopped
3-4 tbsp. red balsamic vinegar
Chilli sauce (optional)

This is a really dark coloured variation on the well-known red onion condiment and goes well with robust grilled fish and also fried fish. When I have produced this it has been for immediate use, so I have no idea what the storage qualities would be like; although properly stored red onion marmalade kept in a fridge may keep for 2 to 3 months. For a slightly different spicy alternative, add a few drops of chilli sauce along with the vinegar. Rice vinegar may also be used for a milder version and has less of a vinegary bite.

• Sweat the onion in a little oil over a low heat until the onion softens, stirring from time to time.

• Then add the sugar and continue cooking until the onion juices have evaporated and it starts to caramelize – about 30 to 40 minutes – but stir occasionally to ensure the mixture does not stick to the pan and burn.

• Add the balsamic vinegar and dulse, stir thoroughly, and allow to cook for another 20 to 30 minutes, adding a splash of water if the mixture appears to be drying out.

SEAWEED DIP / SAUCE

2-3 tbsp. dried dulse, or sea lettuce, finely chopped
¼ cup mayonnaise
¼ cup sour cream
1 tsp. minced shallot
1 tsp. lemon juice
Pepper

This light dip may be used as an addition to a salad or dish containing fish, or even if you are trying to introduce friends to the concept of eating seaweeds without them getting the jitters at the thought of eating some alien form of food. Where using *dried* dulse, use the lemon juice to partly rehydrate the seaweed for a few minutes before mixing with the other ingredients.

• To make the dip, place the first five ingredients in a bowl. Mix, and then add seasoning to taste.

To pep this recipe up it is possible to add touches of Dijon mustard or Tabasco sauce, while the addition of chopped gherkins and capers would put it in the realms of a true tartar sauce.

TUNA KELP SALAD

½-1 cup sugar kelp, raw (finely shredded)
½ cup cucumber, sliced
1 small can tuna flakes
2-3 tsp. light soy sauce
½ tsp. clear honey
1 tsp. white wine vinegar
Lemon juice, splash
1 tbsp. sunflower oil

Since the kelp here is being consumed raw it is important that only the very softest outer frilly border of juvenile sugar kelp specimens is used; the inner crinkly segment of sugar kelp being pretty tough, even when young. Sea lettuce or wakame may also be substituted in this recipe. Where older sugar kelp specimens only are available, then the outer part could be shredded finely and pre-cooked to tenderize it, drained, refreshed in chilled water, before being used as an ingredient.

Alternatively, drop the flaked tuna and transform the other vegetable ingredients into a small accompanying salad garnish to go with a cooked tuna steak.

As yet another recipe alternative, cook a fresh mackerel and substitute the flaked flesh for the tuna ingredient.

• Place the young sugar kelp and sliced cucumber in a bowl.

• Drain the canned tuna (if in oil, then that could substitute for the sunflower oil listed), and add to the bowl.

• Mix all the dressing ingredients together in a small dish, drizzle over the salad, toss and serve.

SUGAR KELP SALAD

½-1 cup sugar kelp
1 small red pepper
2 inches cucumber, peeled
1 tbsp. rice vinegar
1 tbsp. light soy sauce
Garlic purée, to taste (optional)
Caster sugar, pinch
2-3 tsp. sesame oil

Use the outer border part of a piece of young sugar kelp – in total about 10 cm square of frond. Tender young fronds of sea spaghetti could also substitute. The key thing here is to make sure the sugar kelp frond is tender and young. If the kelp looks in any way to be tough then extended cooking time will be necessary.

• Wash the kelp then pat dry, roll into a sausage shape, and slice into thin strips. Drop the pieces into boiling water and cook for 3 or 4 minutes.

• Meanwhile, de-seed a red pepper, cut into strips lengthways, and place in a bowl.

• Take the seaweed off the cooker, drain, and refresh the strips with cold water. Drain again, and set aside.

• Then cut the peeled cucumber into thick matchsticks, and add these to the sliced pepper.

• Pat the seaweed dry on kitchen paper and add to the bowl.

• Next, make up a dressing with the remaining ingredients, mix well, and drizzle over the vegetables.

• Fold everything through using a fork, and decorate with a sprinkling of sesame seeds if so wished.

KELP and HOT RICE SALAD

1 cup brown rice, cooked
Piece of young kelp 3 or 4 inches square, finely shredded
½ red pepper, cubed

Olive oil
Rice wine vinegar
Light soy sauce
Garlic, crushed / to taste (optional)

Another simple combination that hardly needs a recipe. If the kelp you have is a little older then add this to the brown rice when cooking it, since the longer cooking time for brown rice will be beneficial for tenderizing the seaweed. Dabberlocks is a really ideal candidate here, or dulse.

• Place the hot, cooked, rice in a bowl. Add the shredded kelp and cubed pepper, and fold in with a fork.

• In a small dish mix the other ingredients for a dressing then drizzle this over the ingredients when serving.

TANGLED RICE SALAD

1 piece of tangle (about 4 inches square) - finely shredded
2¼ cups water
1 cup uncooked brown rice
½-1 cup mixed seaside greens (optional)
1 small spring onion – finely sliced
1 small carrot – grated
1 tsp. ginger – grated
2-3 tbsp. rice wine vinegar
1 tsp. clear honey
1 tbsp. olive oil
Pepper

This is a recipe for dealing with the more firm kelp-type seaweed species, being added to brown rice and utilizing the long cooking period involved with that ingredient.

If you're down on the beach then it would be worth looking for some additional edible wild veggies to add to this recipe, for colour mainly. They will obviously need preparing appropriately and adding at different stages of the recipe – orache (*Atriplex* sp.) and sea beet (*Beta vulgaris maritima*) blanched in boiling water, roughly chopped, and added in the last stages; young sea aster (*Aster tripolium*) leaves either cooked and combined later, or chopped small and combined with the raw salad ingredients; and tender young buck's-horn plantain (*Plantago coronopus*) leaves, also added at the later stages.

• Bring some water to the boil in a heavy-bottomed pan and add the brown rice and shredded kelp.

• Allow to boil for a few minutes then reduce the heat to a simmer and cover. Simmer the rice 20 minutes, or according to pack directions.

• Meanwhile, place the spring onion and carrot in bowl (and any other chosen raw wild ingredient).

• In a separate dish combine the ginger, vinegar, honey and oil. Mix thoroughly and set aside.

• Once the rice is cooked add it to the raw ingredients, along with the vinaigrette, fold with a fork, and serve.

KELP RELISH

Kelp
Soy sauce
Water

Rice wine vinegar (optional)
Lime juice (optional)
Tabasco sauce (optional)

The big thick kelps such as *Laminaria digitata*, but potentially also more mature sugar kelp and dabberlocks are, from my personal perspective on edible seaweeds, pretty indigestible and have a tendency to be tough when compared to sea lettuce, gutweed and that traditional Japanese favourite wakame. The slow cooking process used here is a good method of making the tougher kelps usable. Even so, I would seek out the very youngest specimens and the most tender growth for this recipe – simply because they will require less cooking and be far more palatable.

The way I view this kelp relish is being something akin to the lime pickle which appears as an accompaniment to Indian food (particularly if you use dark soy sauce). In this case, however, the relish is more of an accompaniment to fish, or as an additional item for salads.

The optional vinegar, lime juice and chilli sauce ingredients listed above provide you with three alternative twists to the relish – one tart, one tangy, one spicy. The first time you experiment with this I suggest working on the plain soy sauce version, and then simply trialling the final outcome with vinegar, lime juice and chilli added to taste and see which alternative you prefer.

• Scrape or score the surfaces of the kelp fronds with a small serrated knife, then cut into squares about ½ to ¾-inch wide.

• Place the pieces in a pan and add equal amounts of soy sauce and water so that the seaweed is just covered with liquid. Add the optional flavourings at this point too.

• Bring the contents of the pan to a boil, then reduce to a simmer, cover and cook gently until the seaweed is tender and most of the liquid has evaporated (think of the consistency of lime pickle), adding more warm water from time to time as necessary.

• When done bottle the relish, allow to cool and store in a refrigerator.

SEA LETTUCE and CUCUMBER SALAD

½ cup cucumber, sliced
2-3 light soy sauce
2 tbsp. apple cider vinegar
1 tsp. clear honey
¼ cup sea lettuce
Sesame seeds

More of a salad accompaniment, this recipe can be also made with the tender young fronds of dulse; the purple-red colour of which complements the cucumber green, though I personally rather like to see the two shades of green in the final outcome.

The seaweed may be chopped, shredded, or cut into squares, depending on whatever visual presentation outcome appeals to you. Dulse cut into squares offsets the cucumber rounds, for example.

• In a small pan warm the soy, vinegar and honey, then remove from the heat and chill the mixture in the fridge.

• Meanwhile, peel the cucumber, slice, and place in a bowl.

• Cut, slice, shred or chop the seaweed, add to the cucumber, and fold the ingredients together with a fork.

• Drizzle over the chilled dressing, garnish with sesame seeds, and serve.

SULTANA and SEA LETTUCE SALAD

½-1 cup sea lettuce
¼ cup raisins / sultanas
Vinegar
Sunflower oil
Paprika, pinch
Ground cumin, pinch

• Shred the seaweed, blanche in boiling water for a couple of minutes, then drain and refresh in cold water.

• Drain the seaweed again, squeezing out any excess water, and place in a bowl.

• Add a little hot water to the raisins or sultanas to puff them up, then drain and add to the seaweed.

• Mix a small amount of oil and vinegar for a dressing in a small dish, then whisk in pinches of paprika and cumin with a fork.

• Drizzle the dressing over the combined salad ingredients, mix together well, then serve.

SEAWEED CAESAR SALAD

2 slices white bread, cubed
Garlic purée, to taste
Sunflower / Olive oil
1 cup sea lettuce, torn
Anchovy fillets, roughly chopped
½ fresh orange, juiced

This is not quite the true Caesar salad, which incorporates Parmesan and raw eggs, but a kind of seaweed take on it. Prepared commercial wakame seaweed is an alternative here, while there is the option of using either marinaded white anchovy fillets or the very salty tinned variety. In the case of the orange, I prefer more acidic ones for this, rather than ultra sweet varieties.

• Cube the bread into pieces, about small finger thickness.

• Heat a little oil in a frying pan, stirring a very little garlic purée into the oil, then fry the bread cubes until they are golden brown all over, making sure to stir constantly to prevent the bread from burning.

• Remove from the heat and drain the cubes on paper kitchen towel.

• Place the seaweed in a small dish, then add the fried bread, and sprinkle the chopped anchovy over.

• Drizzle over the squeezed orange juice, and serve.

TOMATO and SEAWEED SALAD

½ cup sea lettuce, sliced
¼ cup gutweed, chopped
6-8 cherry tomatoes, halved
1 small red onion, chopped
1 tbsp. fresh lime juice
Caster sugar, pinch

Rehydrated wakame would also be an alternative here and could be used raw, or cooked as mentioned below, although this is unnecessary providing the wakame is properly rehydrated (in about 4 to 6 minutes).

• Drop the seaweeds into boiling water and cook for 3 or 4 minutes, then remove from the heat, drain, refresh in cold water, drain again and place in a mixing bowl.

• Add the tomatoes, onion, and fold into the seaweed with a fork.

• Make a dressing by dissolving a little sugar in some lime juice, then pour over the seaweed mixture. Serve.

Still on a tomato-seaweed roll, experiment with a **SEAWEED CHUTNEY** in which wakame is used as the seaweed ingredient. Tomatoes and green chilli (tomato purée and green Tabasco can substitute) are blended and added to chopped frying onion, along with pinches of garam masala, ground cumin, and sugar. When these ingredients have cooked for a few minutes add shredded wakame (pre-soaked in water and drained) and then cook for 5 minutes. Allow to cool for use, especially with a spicy fried fish course.

LETTUCE and GUTWEED SALAD

3 or 4 lettuce leaves
¼ cup gutweed, very young
½ small red onion, finely sliced
1 ripe tomato, sliced
2 tsp. rice vinegar
2 tsp. light soy sauce
½ tsp. toasted sesame oil
Small piece stem ginger, pasted
¼ tsp. wasabi paste

Lettuce leaves may be replaced with a much smaller quantity of very tender sea lettuce fronds (remembering that seaweeds are not overly digestible in large quantities). In this case the salad becomes more of a garnish accompaniment.

• Wash the gutweed, and then again, and possibly again – since it has a tendency to hold the finest sand particles – and place in a bowl.

• Slice the lettuce leaves thinly and add to the bowl, along with sliced tomato, and the red onion sliced almost paper thin.

• Place the vinegar, soy, oil, and pasted ginger and wasabi paste in a small dish and mix. The consistency wants to be no thicker than single cream, so add touches more of vinegar and soy as necessary.

• Drizzle the dressing over the bowl ingredients, toss gently, and serve.

SEA SPAGHETTI and BEANSPROUT SALAD

¼-½ cup sea spaghetti, young sprouts
1 cup beansprouts
¼-½ cup cucumber, matchsticks

2-3 tsp. sunflower oil
1-2 tsp. toasted sesame oil
1 tsp. light soy sauce
1-2 tsp. mirin
2 tsp. rice or wine vinegar

• Begin by washing the sea spaghetti, chopping it into two or three inch lengths, then dropping into boiling water.

• Cook at a rapid boil for a couple of minutes, then turn down the heat and simmer for 15 to 20 minutes, or until tender.

• Meanwhile, wash the beansprouts and place in a bowl.

• Next, take a two inch piece of cucumber, remove the green skin, cut into matchsticks and add to the beansprouts.

• Whisk all the other dressing ingredients together in a small dish, then set aside.

• Drain the cooked seaweed, refresh in cold water till chilled and drain again. Add the seaweed to the beansprouts and cucumber.

• Drizzle the dressing over, then toss and mix the vegetable ingredients with a fork.

SEAWEED-BULGUR SALAD

Bulgur wheat
Vegetable stock
2 tbsp. spring onions (green part), finely chopped
1 small red onion, finely chopped
1 medium tomato, chopped
¼-½ cup seaweed, finely chopped
1 tbsp. sunflower oil
2 tbsp. lemon juice

Dulse or one of the tender green seaweed species may be used for this; dulse complementing the reds of the red onion and tomato, or green sea-weeds the spring onion. The bulgur may be used warm, or allowed to cool, depending on your preference for a warm or cold salad.

• Cook enough bulgur wheat, using vegetable stock, for two servings, and place in a bowl.

• Add the spring onion, onion, tomato and seaweed to the bowl and mix everything thoroughly with a fork.

• Make a dressing with the lemon juice and oil, season as required, drizzle over the salad, and serve.

CUCUMBER and SEAWEED SALAD

½ small cucumber
½ cup seaweed
¼ cup cider / rice / white wine vinegar
1 tsp. sesame seeds
2-3 tsp. onion, finely chopped
Ground turmeric, pinch
1 tsp. caster sugar

Use tender seaweed species for this, or pre-cook more robust ones, then refresh in cold water and use as an ingredient.

• Peel the cucumber and cut into 2-inch pieces, then cut in half length-ways, and then slice again into strips.

• Place the cucumber in a small pan with the vinegar and just enough additional water to cover the cucumber pieces.

• Simmer the cucumber over a medium heat until the pieces are softened slightly, then remove with a slotted spoon and allow to cool, and reserve the vinegar liquid in the pan.

• Cut the seaweed into small pieces and place in a serving bowl, then add the cooling cucumber pieces.

• Next, smear a little oil in a frying pan and toast the sesame seeds until they turn golden brown, then turn them out and allow to cool.

• Add a little more oil to the pan and fry the onion until soft.

• Then add a pinch of turmeric, reserved vinegar-water liquid, and sugar. Heat the mixture gently, stirring, until the sugar dissolves.

• Drizzle the dressing over the seaweed and cucumber, then sprinkle the toasted sesame seeds over, and serve.

SEAWEED MAYONNAISE

¼-½ cup mayonnaise
Saffron, small pinch
White wine vinegar
¼-½ cup seaweed, chopped / shredded

Remember those ancient days of the 1970s when vibrant pink prawn cocktail was all the rage? Well here's an alternative seaweed mayo that may be served over lobster, prawns, and shrimps.

The thicker, kelp-like, seaweeds are not appropriate for this recipe, while my personal preference here is the purple species dulse, which has a good taste. For more decorative, presentational, purposes the green sea lettuce and gutweed species could be used, but those rather lack depth in terms of taste.

• Place the mayo in a small mixing bowl.

• Mix a few saffron threads in a little wine vinegar, and allow to soak for 10 to 15 minutes.

• Chop or shred the seaweed, depending on presentational preferences, and set aside.

• Next, add the saffron-vinegar mixture to the mayonnaise and mix in thoroughly.

• Add the seaweed to the mayo and fold through. Spoon over the fish.

INSTANT SEAWEED PICKLE

1 cup seaweed
½ cup shredded carrot (optional)
¼ cup vinegar
1 tbsp. mustard oil
2-3 tsp. caster sugar
Pepper
½ tsp. ground cumin, turmeric
½ tsp. mustard powder
¼-½ tsp. chilli powder

When I first experimented with this recipe on dried seaweed, I left it to marinade for several hours in the vinegar-spice dressing. The end result, with rehydrated dried dulse, was rather soggy. So I now tend to make the pickle with fresh seaweed, mainly the tender green types like sea lettuce, and make this half an hour or so before it is needed. The pickle works well with a spicy fish curry, or similar. Or just use it as an unusual condiment to go with salad. Although untried at the moment, it would be interesting to see how wakame responds to similar treatment.

Mustard oil may often be found in Asian stores in the UK, but in the U.S. the oil is on the health blacklist and recommended for external use only. However, mustard oil is used extensively on the Indian sub-continent in domestic kitchens. Should you feel uncomfortable about the health risks use sunflower or coconut oil as alternatives. The affinity of carrot with seaweed sees the carrot ingredient here as an optional extra for you to experiment with.

• Begin by drying the seaweed with paper towel to remove surface moisture, then cut, chop or shred, as preferred, and place in a small bowl.

• Mix the vinegar with the sugar until the latter is dissolved, then add the oil and mix in the remaining spice ingredients (add a little more or less of any item to personal preference).

• Pour the marinade over the seaweed and toss with a fork.

• Cover with cling film and place in a refrigerator till needed, but uncover the seaweed from time to time and turn with a fork.

VEGETABLES

EGGY SEAWEED

½ cup sea lettuce, chopped
3 medium eggs, beaten
Water
1-2 tsp. sunflower oil.
1-2 tsp. light soy sauce
Salt & pepper

This mixture may be prepared like scrambled egg, or cooked and served as an omelette-type item.

• Beat the eggs in a bowl, then mix in a touch of cold water, and set aside.

• Chop young sea lettuce finely – although finely shredding is possible too – add to the egg-water mixture and stir thoroughly.

• Mix the oil and soy sauce then place in a heated skillet, and swirl around. When hot enough fry or scramble the eggs in the hot oil-soy mixture. Season to taste, and serve.

SQUASH and SUGAR KELP

1 cup – butternut squash, sliced
½-1 cup sugar kelp, shredded
½ cup water
1 tbsp. rice wine / mirin
2 tbsp. light soy sauce
Bonito flakes

Although this is designed as a vegetable side dish, by upping the water content it could be transformed into a broth or soup, and then freshly cooked fish of some description (tuna or mackerel, for example) flaked into the broth in place of the bonito flakes. Bonito flakes are, incidentally, dried tuna flakes, and may be found in some of the larger Oriental and Asian supermarkets as well as from online sources.

Only use the outer frilly boundary layer of a young sugar kelp frond for this recipe. The inner, central part of the fronds, will not cook properly in the time allocated.

• Place the all the ingredients, with the exception of the bonito flakes, into a small, heavy-bottomed pan (ideally cast iron) with a close fitting lid.

• Stir the ingredients well, bring to the boil for 2 or 3 minutes, then cover the pan and turn the heat down really low.

• Cook for 30 minutes and then check moisture levels, season to taste, and re-cover the pan.

• Turn the heat off and allow the residual pan heat to finish off cooking the mixture.

• Serve with flaked bonito sprinkled over.

SLOW SIMMERED SEA SPAGHETTI

½-1 cup sea spaghetti, young sprouts
2 or 3 runner or string beans
2 or 3 shitake or chestnut mushrooms
½ cup vegetable stock
2 tbsp. rice wine / mirin
1-2 tsp. sunflower oil
1-2 tsp. caster sugar
1 tbsp. soy sauce

For this I use the young springtime shoots, or growth, of sea spaghetti, otherwise known as thongweed. The lighter green shoots of the young plants are far superior in texture and taste to the later, darker, growth.

• Begin by cutting the washed sea spaghetti fronds into pieces three or four inches long. Set aside.

• Next, slice the beans into long slivers – about enough to provide about ½ to 1 cup of vegetable. Slice the mushrooms thinly, too.

• Place the stock, mirin, sugar and a little oil in a small, heavy-bottomed, pan. Bring to the boil and add the sea spaghetti, cook for a few minutes, then turn down to a medium heat.

• Simmer for about 5 minutes more, then add the beans, mushrooms and soy sauce.

• Raise the heat briefly until the liquid reaches boiling point, then lower to medium, cover with a lid, and simmer for about 10 to 15 minutes, or until the beans are done.

SEA SPAGHETTI and CARROTS

2 or 3 small carrots, peeled
¼-½ cup young sea spaghetti tips
1-2 tbsp. light soy sauce
1-2 tsp. ginger root, grated

In Japan the seaweed called hijiki is often teamed up with carrots, and this recipe is really a European take on that ingredient-pairing concept.

• Begin by halving the carrots lengthways, then quartering each section so you end up with roughly finger-size pieces. Baby carrots may be used whole, or halved depending on size.

• Next, place the seaweed on the bottom of a small pan and layer the carrot pieces on top.

• Mix the soy sauce and grated ginger with a little water and add to the pan.

• Now add just enough water to cover the vegetables.

• Bring to the boil for a couple of minutes then reduce the heat to low, cover, and cook till the carrots are almost tender (add a touch more water as necessary).

• When almost done, remove the cover and allow the carrots to continue cooking until the water has all but evaporated.

LOTUS ROOT and SEAWEED

½ cup tinned lotus root
½ cup seaweed – sea lettuce, sugar kelp
Sunflower oil
Sesame oil
2 tbsp. rice vinegar
1 tbsp. water
2 tsp. light soy sauce
1 tsp. sugar
1 tsp. sesame seeds, toasted (optional)

This recipe is for a side dish or salad item. While ingredients such as mirin and rice vinegar may often be found in high street supermarkets you will almost certainly need to venture into a Chinese supermarket, or similar, to find lotus roots which have a lovely crunchy texture. If you happen to reside in London then the stores in Chinatown offer numerous dried and canned forms of lotus root.

• Depending on your lotus root source, peel and thinly slice the root and soak in acidified water for 10 minutes (use a splash of the rice vinegar).

• Meanwhile, slice the seaweed of choice and drop into boiling water for 5 minutes in the case of sea lettuce, or 10 to 15 minutes for young sugar kelp fronds. Drain, and set aside.

• In a small dish mix the vinegar, water, soy sauce and sugar, until the sugar is dissolved.

• Next, drain the lotus slices, and pat dry.

• Put a little of each oil into a frying pan over a medium heat and fry the lotus slices until they start to soften.

• Reduce the heat, then add the vinegar mixture and stir through. Cook for a couple of minutes then add the seaweed and gently stir-fry so that all the ingredients are coated with the sauce mixture.

• Sprinkle the sesame seeds over, if using, and serve.

SEA LETTUCE QUICHE, KEDGEREE, PAELLA and STUFFED

Neither quiche nor kedgeree should require much explanation so there are no recipes below. Just follow any basic spinach-like quiche recipe you might find in a cookbook, even to the extent of buying pre-made flan cases (see page 90), and use chopped sea lettuce as the vegetable ingredient.

Because of the pastry nature of the dish it is best to dry the sea lettuce on kitchen paper towel before mixing with the beaten egg. This reduces excess moisture which could make the pastry soggy.

Adding a bit of flaked mackerel to the mix, small shrimps, or even some chopped smoked salmon, provides further seafood angles.

As for kedgeree, follow any basic kedgeree cooking method, but use sea lettuce to replace the peas, and flaked mackerel as the fish ingredient. Personally, I prefer to drop the egg ingredient when using this combination, though you might keep it. The thing is to explore the kedgeree concept.

Although purple laver is not quite so visually attractive, it may also be used as a substitute for sea lettuce if finely shredded, as could chopped gutweed, and wakame too.

In the case of paella, follow the basic recipe available to you and then introduce seaweed at the appropriate point in the recipe – more tender species such as sea lettuce towards the end, and more robust seaweed species near the beginning of the cooking period. Similarly, a mushroom risotto with a little tender seaweed added is another interesting culinary avenue to explore for anyone with a penchant for Italian cuisine or savoury rice dishes.

In all the instances above a sprinkling of crumbled laver or 'sea spice' (dried seaweed finely crushed to the consistency of table salt) adds another flavour embellishment.

For the stuffed sea lettuce leaves, select larger fronds then stuff with some mashed tinned anchovy fillets to which a small slug of rice or white wine vinegar has been added. Take spoonfuls of the anchovy mash and a little cooked white rice, place in the centre of a sea lettuce frond and wrap into a bundle (if necessary use a cocktail stick to hold the bundle in shape). Then simply steam the bundles for 5 minutes and serve.

Virtually any white sea fish can be similarly packaged in sea lettuce fronds and steamed.

TOMATO and SEAWEED RICE

1 medium / small onion, sliced
Sunflower oil
½ tsp. ginger root, minced
Ground turmeric, large pinch
Chilli powder, pinch
1 large tomato, chopped
1 cup basmati rice
2 cups water
¼-½ cup dulse, chopped or shredded

Although other domestic seaweeds could be used for this, even wakame, I personally think the purple-red of the dulse visually complements the red of the tomato.

• Stir-fry the onion in a little oil until just turning golden brown, then stir in the ginger, turmeric and chilli powder and cook for a further minute.

• Add the tomato and continue stir-frying for 5 minutes.

• Next, combine the rice to the onion-tomato mixture and gently stir to distribute evenly. Add the water and stir in, then cover and cook over a low heat until the rice is done.

• Meanwhile, rehydrate the dulse for a few minutes in water, then drain, press out as much water as possible and separate the pieces. Set aside.

• When the rice is done add the dulse and fold into the rice with a fork. Allow to warm through for 5 minutes then serve.

SEA LETTUCE and RICE

White rice
Sea lettuce
Sesame oil, splash
Light soy sauce, slug
Sesame seeds, pinch

Another recipe which doesn't really require a method, being essentially sea lettuce added to cooked white rice, although I frequently use commercially available wakame for this as it rehydrates in only a few minutes.

While your rice is cooking to perfection...

• Make a small amount of marinade made with sesame oil, sesame seeds, and soy sauce.

• Rub washed sea lettuce leaves with this mixture and put the leaves in a pile on a piece of kitchen foil with any remaining marinade.

• Make an envelope of the foil and place in a pre-heated moderate oven (180°C) and bake for about 10 minutes.

• Remove from the oven, allow to cool to handling temperature, then shred.

• Sprinkle the lettuce greens on your cooked rice – or even fold into the rice. That's really down to presentational goals.

Another very simple seaweed-rice dish you may like to experiment with is a **SEAWEED JOLOFF** rice; joloff having its origins in African cuisine. Drop the garlic if you wish, but keep the onions, green chilli and tomato purée, then add dried wakame pieces when the stock is added to cook the rice.

SEAWEED COUSCOUS

¼-½ cup dried seaweed, crumbled
Couscous
Vegetable stock
Extra hot water
Lemon juice
Sesame oil
1-2 tbsp. light soy sauce
1-2 tbsp. white wine / cider vinegar

To my mind couscous is one of those ingredients which always seems to take a lot of effort to make inspiring eating. When I first experimented with this recipe, which may be served alongside a fish dish – spicy, for example – I used imported dried wakame foraged from my local Asian supermarket. Other similar native dried European seaweeds could also substitute, but they do need to be crumbled from pieces of tender frond. Dried kelps would not be much use here unless pre-cooked and then added to the recipe.

• Begin by measuring out enough dry couscous for 2 servings according to pack directions, and similarly follow pack directions for the volume of vegetable stock.

• Next, crumble the dry seaweed, add to the couscous in a bowl, and mix thoroughly. The crumbled seaweed pieces want to be about tea-leaf size.

• Stir the boiling vegetable stock into the bowl, and then top up with a little more boiling water until the mixture is slightly wet (allows for liquid adsorbtion by the dry seaweed). Then cover with cling film and leave for 5 to 10 minutes.

• Meanwhile, make a dressing with the lemon juice, light soy sauce, a little sesame oil, and a small amount of vinegar – adjusting to personal taste.

• Next, remove the cling film and check the couscous tenderness (if still slightly underdone flash in a microwave for a few seconds).

• Drizzle the dressing over the couscous-seaweed mixture and mix thoroughly. Serve heaped, or in timbale form with a fish dish.

MUSHROOM, SEAWEED and BULGUR PATTIES

1 cup reconstituted bulgur wheat
2 tbsp. laver or dulse, finely chopped
Ground cumin, pinch
½ tsp. mustard (optional)
½ cup mushrooms, very finely sliced
Sunflower oil

The end product of this experimental recipe are small flat patties of bulgur which are fragile to handle, so make the patties small. For less fragile patties beaten egg may be added to the bulgur as a binder. Pressing the mixture into small moulds then chilling for 20 minutes also helps.

• Reconstitute enough bulgur wheat for 2 servings according to the pack directions, place in a bowl and allow to cool for a few minutes.

• Add the chopped seaweed and mix thoroughly.

• Next, blend the mixture with a hand blender – or transfer to a dedicated blender – and whiz until something akin to a partial paste is formed (add touches of more water to achieve a mouldable consistence, but do not make the mixture wet).

• Next, stir in the finely sliced mushrooms, mustard (if using), and mix well.

• Heat a little oil in a non-stick frying pan (definitely the best option).

• Take heaped tablespoons of the mixture, drop into the pan and flatten out with the back of the spoon into patties of about pencil-thickness.

• Fry the patties on each side for about 5 or 6 minutes, using a spatula or fish slice to carefully turn them over. Since the patties are fragile avoid moving them unnecessarily during frying.

• Cook until golden brown and crisp on the outside.

SEAWEED BULGUR PILAF

1 cup bulgur wheat
Butter
1 cup vegetable (or beef) stock
Seaweed
Salt and pepper
Flaked cooked fish, prawns or shrimps (optional)

The outcome of this recipe can be presented either as a hot meal, or it could be chilled and served up as a salad. If not opting to add fish then it may also be eaten as an accompaniment to fish, while I sometimes have this pilaf on its own (as in, without fish) for breakfast instead of toast or porridge. In other variations I add chopped tomato and shredded carrot.

A tender seaweed such as sea lettuce, dulse, young dabberlocks or sugar kelp is required. If using older or larger seaweeds then it would be best to pre-cook or par-boil them till tender, then add to the bulgur.

• Cut your selected seaweed into fork-size pieces and set aside.

• Melt a large knob of butter in a heavy-bottomed pan and sauté the bulgur for a few minutes, stirring the mixture moving to prevent it from burning.

• Next, heat the stock and then add it to the wheat, along with the seaweed. Mix well together.

• Then fold in your cooked fish ingredient with a fork, cover, and cook over a low heat until the stock is absorbed (about 20 minutes).

• Season as required, although I sometimes simply drizzle over a little light soy sauce.

SOYA MINCE and SEAWEED

½-1 cup young sea spaghetti
Soya mince
1 small-medium carrot, finely chopped
Spring onion, thinly sliced (optional)
½ tbsp. sesame oil
½ tbsp. mirin
Caster sugar, pinch
1-2 tbsp. light soy sauce

Soya mince is available from high street supermarkets for vegetarian meals such as faux bolognese. However it has a place in seaweed dishes. Here the seaweed wants to be the very youngest new spring growth since this requires very little cooking time – almost being used as a blanched semi-raw ingredient.

• Begin by making up enough reconstituted soya mince for 2 servings, according to pack instructions.

• Meanwhile, chop the sea spaghetti into finger width lengths, boil in water for 5 minutes, drain, and set aside.

• Next, finely chop or matchstick the carrot and fry gently in a little vegetable oil until the carrot begins to soften. If opting for spring onion, add this about 5 minutes after starting to cook the carrot.

• Add the cooked sea spaghetti to the pan, and stir in. Turn the heat low.

• Add the prepared soya mince to the pan and mix everything together thoroughly. Cover the pan and cook for 5 to 10 minutes.

• Make a dressing with the remaining ingredients, and place in a sauce dish.

• Serve the soya-seaweed mince with the dressing drizzled over.

DABBERLOCKS and TOFU

½-1 cup dabberlocks
2-3 sliced tofu cubes
½ tbsp. sesame oil
¼ cup carrot, shredded
1 tbsp. mirin
1 tbsp. light soy sauce
Salt and pepper

• Cut a young dabberlocks frond (the midrib removed) into fork-size pieces and fry gently in the oil.

• Then add the sliced tofu and cook for a couple of minutes.

• Remove both from the pan and set aside.

• Next, add the shredded carrot to the pan and cook over a medium heat until it begins to soften.

• Return the seaweed and tofu to the pan, then add mirin and soy sauce, stir well and cover.

• Simmer gently until the vegetables are tender (adding a splash of water or vegetable stock if the mixture appears to be drying, or adding even more liquid to make this recipe more broth-like).

• Season to taste as required, and serve.

FRIED TOFU and SEAWEED

4 oz firm tofu
Sunflower oil
Toasted sesame oil
½-¾ cup gutweed
2 tbsp. light soy sauce
2 tbsp. mirin
2 tbsp. sweet sherry
Chilli powder / flakes, pinch (optional)

There are two ways of presenting the tofu in this side dish recipe – either sliced, or cubed. Personally I think the visual presentation looks better when sliced, but that's down to you on the day.

If not using sweet sherry, use the dry variety and dissolve a little caster sugar in the sauce mixture.

• Begin by washing the gutweed (and a couple of times more to remove any traces of fine sand), drain, and then chop into 1 to 2-inch lengths. Set aside.

• Next, heat a good slug of the oils in a frying pan – just enough to lubricate the bottom of the frying pan.

• When very hot, add the tofu block or cubes and fry until golden brown, turning the tofu so it is golden and the sides crispy. When done, remove the tofu with a slotted spoon and allow to cool on kitchen paper.

• Meanwhile, in a small dish mix the soy, mirin and sherry, and add a pinch of chilli. Set aside.

• When sufficiently cool to handle slice the tofu into pencil thickness pieces, and place in a serving dish.

• Distribute the gutweed across the tofu.

• Next, put the frying pan back over the heat, and heat the sauce mixture for a couple of minutes.

• Finally, pour the hot sauce over the tofu-gutweed and gently turn the mixture with a fork to better distribute the sauce then serve.

SEAWEED, TOFU and SPLIT PEAS

1 cup yellow split peas, cooked
½ cup tofu, cubed
Sunflower oil
Black mustard seeds, good pinch
¼ tsp. turmeric
¼ tsp. cumin
Pepper
¼-½ cup seaweed, sliced, shredded or chopped

This is another of those side dish recipes where the seaweed species may be varied, according to season, availability, and age. For tougher specimens they will need to be pre-cooked and then added to the split peas, while softer and more tender species such as sea lettuce, gutweed, or even wakame, may be added really without any pre-cooking.

• Begin by heating a little oil in a frying pan and frying the tofu pieces till they take on a bit of golden colour. Then remove from the pan with a slotted spoon and set aside.

• Add a little more oil to the pan (if required) and fry some mustard seeds until they start to sputter.

• Next, add the split peas, then the spices and pepper seasoning, and stir-fry for several minutes.

• Add the seaweed plus a splash of water and continue stir-frying for 7 or 8 minutes over a medium heat.

• Return the tofu to the pan, and cook for another minute or two until the tofu is warmed through.

PASTA with DULSE

Conchiglie or penne pasta
Dried dulse
Pine kernels
Garlic, crushed / to taste (optional)
Pesto sauce
Parmesan, grated or shavings
Pepper

• Begin by soaking the dulse in a bowl of water for about 5 to 10 minutes to soften, then remove from the water with a slotted spoon and cut the dulse into strips and set aside (reserve a little of the soaking water to add to the sauce).

• Next, begin cooking the pasta in lightly salted water and continue to cook until al dente.

• Meanwhile, lightly fry the pine kernels for a couple of minutes, then add the crushed garlic to the pan. Continue cooking until the garlic is softened, but not browned.

• Stir in a few spoons of green pesto sauce and cook for a minute.

• Add the dulse strips to the pan and cook over a moderate heat for 5 minutes or so (adding a little of the reserved soaking water to create a sauce which coats the back of a spoon), and season as required.

• Drain the pasta and then either serve with the sauce spooned over, or add to the sauce ingredients in the pan and thoroughly coat with the sauce, serving with Parmesan sprinkled over.

Something you my like to experiment with is a **SEAWEED PESTO** made from blended sea lettuce fronds, and then flavoured with chilli, fish sauce, or similar sorts of flavours. It is a bit of a gimmick to be truthful but kind of goes with fish dishes and, potentially, pasta, where you want a taste of the sea. This pesto also allows you to play a culinary sleight of hand on the plate as it has the appearance of wasabi paste yet tastes nothing like it.

If you do decide to give it a try make sure to chop the sea lettuce fronds into small bits before you blend them, since sheets of the seaweed can become knotted round the cutting blades otherwise. This is also a good way to use up raggedy sea lettuce fronds unfit for plate presentation.

SEAWEED and PEA CAKES

1½-2 cups mashed potato
1 small shallot, minced
1-2 tbsp. frozen peas
¼-½ cup seaweed
1 tsp. finely chopped green chilli
1 tsp. garam masala
½ tsp. ground turmeric
Sunflower oil
Salt and pepper

An accompaniment to a fish dish, this recipe can utilize many seaweed species, although tough species will require chopping or shredding and pre-cooking before being incorporated within the potato. Delicate seaweeds such as gutweed and sea lettuce present little problem, as will wakame.

• Place the mashed potato in a bowl.

• Cook the peas in a little water till tender, then drain well and add to the mash.

• Add the seaweed, onion and spices to the bowl and mix through with a fork. Add seasoning as required.

• Take heaped tablespoons of the mixture and form into flat patties.

• Put some oil in the bottom of a frying pan and carefully fry the patties at a medium heat for about 5 minutes on each side, or until golden. Handle carefully as the patties are quite fragile.

POTATO and SEAWEED

No recipes here, but some suggestions rather, on combining seaweed with humble spuds. These go particularly well as a vegetable alongside fish; whether served as a complementary item in a starter, or with a more substantial main fish course.

[1] If you have sliced sautéd potatoes then sprinkle over some minced, dried, dulse before serving.

[2] Boiled new potatoes, or boiled cubed larger ones, can be sprinkled with finely chopped sea lettuce, dulse or young sugar kelp, or any combination of these. In relation to that last point, try dusting potatoes with the so-called seaweed salt / sea spice (ground dried seaweed).

Making your own seaweed salt / sea spice by grinding fragments of dried seaweed lurking in the store cupboard is a good way of using them up. Sautéd potatoes may also be sprinkled with the 'salt' for a different twist.

[3] Where mashed potato is being served, mix chopped sea lettuce or gutweed into the mash. Of course the mash could then be used to make croquettes. Dried sea lettuce and laver also make good seaweed condiments to potato, when dried, crushed, and sprinkled over.

[4] A seaweed and potato tortilla / frittata is also another possibility – add some fish ingredient if you wish to give it more of a seafood twist.

[5] A tasty potato-seaweed fry-up is possible too, using wakame or similar fine seaweed. The soaked, drained, seaweed is added to fried cubed potato, and sliced onion, which have been fried separately. All the ingredients are folded together then cooked with beaten egg – scrambled fricasée-like – then served with fried bread croutons previously prepared.

[6] A play on the Indian side dish *sag aloo* is possible too, and served with a fish or shellfish curry. Wakame, rehydrated in hot water and drained, is added to fried cubed or sliced potato pieces dusted with flaked chilli and garam masala.

FRIED SEAWEED

When frying any seaweed it is a good idea to run a small test batch first since the outcome depends on the quality of frond growth, seaweed species, as well as oil temperature. Young kelps crisp up in 20 to 30 seconds while fine gutweeds may take just 10 seconds and are burnt to cinders if cooked much longer. We are, incidentally, talking about cooking fresh not dried seaweed here. Dried seaweed will require re-hydration first and in both cases fronds need patting dry before frying, as hot oil and water do not mix. Anyway, my suggestion is to test fry a sample before committing the whole lot to your deep fryer, and keeping a safe distance from the fryer as you submerge the damp sea-weed in the oil. And watch the cooking time as scorched seaweed tastes awful.

Kelp Chips

Frying kelp is a cooking method I keep reserved for older, but not too old, fronds. Simply slice larger kelp fronds into pencil thickness 'chip' sizes then deep-fry them as you would potato chips. If they are cooked to perfection the end result is crunchy and slightly porous in texture, almost like a pork scratching without the fat. They are rather fun to serve with Thai sweet chilli sauce as a dip. With tomato ketchup – heaven forbid – even youngsters may be enticed to give seaweed a try.

Deep-fried Sea Spaghetti / Thongweed

Deep-frying sea spaghetti is my personal answer to older fronds which, in my view, have an awful texture. The fronds may be cut into small matchstick size lengths up to about six inches long. Pat them dry and deep fry. Being quite thin they take about 10 to 15 seconds to cook, sometimes longer, though by a minute they are generally overcooked and scorched. I serve these fried with a dipping sauce of blended prawns and tomato purée, thinned with a little oil or stock.

Gutweed

Deep-frying gutweed needs to be done with some caution as the fronds of different species contain trapped air pockets of varying sizes which can explode when immersed in the deep fryer. *Enteromorpha linza* and *compressa* are best since the air pockets are tiny, while I would not use the true gutweed (*E. intestinalis*) unless you have made serious attempts to expel the air in the bladders. Toss the fried gutweed with a few drops of oyster sauce before serving.

FISH

GRILLED OYSTERS and SEAWEED

Oysters
Dulse and/or sea lettuce
Breadcrumbs
Olive oil

Call me a culinary Philistine but I am not the world's greatest admirer of raw oysters, preferring them cooked as in this recipe. For this recipe I prefer a light or mild olive oil rather than an extra virgin, but that is a personal taste issue, while a little melted butter is another alternative if calories or cholesterol are not a dietary issue. Although untried, this might possibly work with larger sized mussels, perhaps with a little garlic added to the breadcrumb mixture.

• Begin by pre-heating the grill.

• Next, mince a small amount of dulse or sea lettuce, or both combined. The chopped size wants to be something akin to mint leaves prepared for mint sauce.

• Place the seaweed mince in a small bowl and add an equivalent amount of breadcrumbs. Mix well.

• Shuck the oysters, keeping them in a half shell.

• Sprinkle the seaweed-breadcrumb mixture over each oyster evenly, then drizzle with a little oil.

• Place under the grill and cook for 2 to 3 minutes, or until the oysters are cooked through.

FISH and SEAWEED PUDDING

2 cups fish meat, minced
1 small tin of crab meat
1 small plaice fillet
½ cup cooked peas
½ cup seaweed, chopped / shredded

Although the crab can be tinned the other fish ingredients here need to be fresh, otherwise the 'pudding' will not hold together. Potentially this recipe could be used for most pelagic fish, whether you are using up scraps sticking to bones, or prime fillet meat.

Virtually any seaweed may be used too, though the thicker species will need a little pre-cooking to soften them. In preference, I shred seaweed for this recipe as I think the presentational outcome is more interesting than the 'bitty' visual appearance of finely chopped seaweed.

• Begin by mincing whatever white fish you decide to use (hand process in preference to blending with a mixer), and place in a mixing bowl.

• Drain the crab meat and place in another mixing bowl.

• Next, cut the plaice fillet into fork-size pieces. Set aside.

• Mix in the peas and seaweed, then add these to the minced fish and crab meat and fold through with a fork.

• Next, butter or lightly oil a suitable size mould, then place a finger-thick layer of the minced fish mixture on the bottom of the mould.

• Place pieces of cut fillet on top, then fill the remainder of the mould with fish-pea mixture. (If you have too many fillet pieces, simply create a layered 'pudding').

• Cover the mould with foil, and tie down with kitchen string.

• Put a large pan on the hob, place the mould in the centre and fill the pan with hot water – within a couple of finger widths from the mould rim (alternatively use a proper steamer pan).

• Bring the water to a gently rolling boil, then cover the pan and cook for 30 to 40 minutes.

SEAWEED STUFFED ONIONS

4 medium red onions
½-1 cup fresh fish meat
1-2 tbsp. seaweed, chopped
1 slice white bread, crumbed
1 hard-boiled egg yolk
Salt and pepper
White wine
1 tbsp. cream
Butter

• Cut the tops off the onions, and make a small cut across the root end to help it stand level.

• Then hollow out each onion until the wall is about ¼-inch thick.

• Mince, or finely chop, about 1 tbsp. of the removed onion centres, and set aside.

• Next, chop the fish finely and place in a mixing bowl, and mix in the crumbed bread (reserving about 1 tbsp. of the crumbs), the chopped onion and seaweed.

• Mash the egg yolk with a fork and combine with the fish-egg-seaweed mixture.

• Dribble over a little white wine and the cream, then mix thoroughly and stuff the onions with the mixture.

• Sprinkle the reserved breadcrumbs over the top hole and add a small pat of butter.

• Bake in a moderately-hot oven (190°C) for 30 to 40 minutes.

While on the subject of *stuffing*, another something you may like to try is stuffing large fish fillets, fish steaks, or even whole fish with a mixture of finely chopped wakame and minced prawns or shrimps, with or without the addition of chilli.

SHRIMPS and SEAWEED

1 cup rehydrated dried shrimps
1 large tomato, skinned
1 small shallot, chopped
Sunflower oil
2 cups cooked haricot / canellini beans
½-1 cup seaweed

From personal knowledge dried shrimps (not prawns) may usually be obtained from Chinese and Asian supermarkets in London, though I am uncertain whether high street supermarket chains stock this ingredient.

My seaweed of choice here is one of the milder tasting ones such as sea lettuce or gutweed. Pre-cooked shredded sugar kelp is another alternative which you could potentially add in its raw state when cooking the shallot-tomato pulp. And one imagines that commercially available arame might be a substitute although the brown-black stringy fronds could look a tad unsightly in terms of presentation. The more tender seaweeds need adding towards the back end of the recipe.

• Soak the dried shrimps in a little warm water for 10 to 15 minutes.

• Meanwhile, fry the shallot and tomato in a little oil until they begin to pulp, then stir in the garlic purée, and add some of the shrimp soaking water (add shredded sugar kelp at this point too, if using). Simmer until a thick sauce forms.

• Put the cooked beans in a separate pan, with the tender seaweed pieces, rehydrated shrimps and the remainder of the soaking liquid, plus a cup of water.

• Bring to the boil briefly, then stir in the tomato-shallot mixture. Allow to come to the boil again then turn down the heat, cover, simmer for 10 minutes and serve.

CRUSTED HADDOCK

¼ cup seaweed, finely chopped
½-1 cup fresh white breadcrumbs
2 haddock fillets, skinless
½-1 tsp. garlic purée (optional)
Olive oil

The fresh seaweed here wants to be one of the more robust flavoured ones, such as dulse, rather than mild sea lettuce or gutweed. The cooking method, however, is very simple. If using dried seaweed it is important to rehydrate this since the dish is baked in the oven and dried seaweed may well scorch under such cooking conditions.

• Dry the fillets with a piece of kitchen paper then place in a lightly oiled baking dish large enough to hold the fillets.

• Place the seaweed in a bowl, and if opting for garlic add that now and mix in with a fork.

• Add breadcrumbs to the bowl and mix in, and then a little olive oil. Mix everything thoroughly.

• Spoon the mixture evenly over the fillets and press lightly down.

• Bake in a pre-heated moderate oven (180°C) for about 20 to 25 minutes or until the fish is cooked through. [Lightly cover with a piece of aluminium foil should the seaweed topping appear to start scorching.]

HADDOCK and SEAWEED CRUMBLE

1-2 cups cooked haddock meat, flaked
½-1 cup dabberlocks, leafy part
1 small onion, chopped
1 medium potato, diced
1 carrot, diced
Sunflower oil
3 tbsp. butter
3 tbsp. plain flour
¼ cup vegetable stock
Cream
Cayenne

1 cup plain flour
½ cup butter

- Cut the dabberlocks into fork-size pieces and boil in water for about 5 minutes. Then remove from the heat, drain, and set aside.

- Meanwhile, lightly oil a suitably sized ovenproof dish, and distribute the cooked fish over the bottom.

- Next, sweat the potato, onion and carrot in a little oil for 2 or 3 minutes, then cover the pan and cook until just softened. Distribute the cooked vegetables over the flaked fish.

- Layer the cooked dabberlocks over the vegetables.

- Melt the butter in a small pan, stir in the flour and cook for a minute, stirring continuously.

- Warm the stock and add to the pan, stirring to ensure a smooth sauce develops. Then add a little cream and stir in. Distribute the sauce evenly over the other ingredients in the ovenproof dish, and add a touch of cayenne for seasoning.

- Make the crumble mixture by rubbing the butter into the flour in a bowl until the texture resembles breadcrumbs. Sprinkle this over the ingredients in the ovenproof dish and place in a pre-heated, moderately-hot oven (200°C), and bake for about 20 minutes.

SALMON and SEAWEED QUICHE

9-inch (savoury) flan case
¼-½ cup smoked salmon, roughly chopped
½ cup sea lettuce or gutweed, chopped
4 medium eggs
½ cup milk
½ cup cream

Years ago, before wild food became fashionable, I remember a food writer from The Times popping along to see what I got up to with wild foods. Being asked on that occasion to rustle up something exotic or unusual I opted to make nettle and wild garlic (ramsons – *Allium ursinum*) quiche tartlets using a largely acorn-based pastry. Here's something not quite so exotic, but still unusual. It is also an interesting way to get folks unfamiliar with eating seaweed to try this novel food in a more familiar form – as a quiche.

This recipe is really for 4 people, unless you can procure (or make) smaller pre-prepared flan cases from a supermarket.

• Start by partially blind-baking the flan case as per pack timings.

• Meanwhile, beat the eggs, milk and cream in a bowl.

• When partially baked remove the flan from the oven and allow to cool briefly.

• Next, distribute the smoked salmon and chopped seaweed evenly over the base of the baked case.

• Give the beaten egg mixture a quick stir then pour over the ingredients in the flan case.

• Place in a pre-heated moderate oven (180°C) and bake for about 30 to 40 minutes, or until the mixture is set and the pastry golden brown.

• Serve with a little flaked, dried, seaweed spinkled over as a garnish.

GUTWEED FISH CAKES

½ cup cooked white fish, flaked
½ cup mashed potato
1 tsp. minced onion
Gutweed, roughly chopped
Pepper, pinch
1 small size egg, beaten
Breadcrumbs
Butter or oil

With this recipe I like to keep some texture to the mixed ingredients, so I fold the contents rather than mash them together. Also, the egg is added in just sufficient quantity to moisten the mass, not create liquid gloop which will not hold together. You can use several or more table-spoons of the seaweed as you will. The breadcrumbs provide a barrier against the seaweed 'catching' when fried.

• Put the main ingredients in a bowl and add half of the beaten egg. Mix everything well, adding more egg as required (the mixture doesn't want to slough on standing but be reasonably firm).

• Then make up faggot-sized portions of the mixture, flatten them into cakes, and then breadcrumb them.

• Heat some oil in a pan and shallow-fry the fishcakes for 4 or 5 minutes on each side or until golden brown.

SEAWEED and CUCUMBER CUPS

Cucumber
Rice vinegar
Caster sugar
¼-½ cup seaweed, finely chopped
¼-½ cup cooked anchovy, mackerel or sardine
1 tsp. grated ginger root
Light soy sauce

This recipe creates a small salad, or side dish, rather than a main course. Assuming an individual could eat three or four of the cucumber 'cups' you will need a piece of cucumber 6 to 8 inches long.

For the seaweed input use sea lettuce, gutweed or pre-cooked sections of dabberlocks or young sugar kelp frond. The anchovies want to be the marinaded-in-oil type, rather than the salty dried ingredient, but if these are unavailable switch to *fresh* mackerel or sardine. Canned supermarket mackerel or sardines really don't do justice to the recipe.

• Begin by cutting the cucumber into 1-inch long pieces, then scoop out the centres leaving about ¼-inch thickness for the base and walls.

• Place the cucumber in a bowl that will tightly fit the pieces, then add enough rice vinegar to just cover the sections. Sprinkle a little sugar over and gently rock the bowl to dissolve the sugar crystals. Leave to marinade until required.

• Meanwhile, place the fish in a bowl and roughly mash with a fork.

• Add the prepared seaweed and fold into the fish.

• In a small dish mix the ginger root with a little soy sauce, plus a small spoonful or two of the vinegar-sugar marinade.

• Add the liquid to the anchovy-seaweed mixture and mix thoroughly.

• Next, drain the cucumber 'cups' and fill with the anchovy mixture. Serve.

SEA BASS with SEAWEED

2 sea bass fillets
1 red shallot, finely chopped
1 small red pepper, sliced
Garlic purée, to taste
½-1 cup tinned baby clams
1 large tomato, de-seeded and chopped
½ cup white wine
1½ cups vegetable stock
¼-½ cup dried laver, finely crumbled
Sunflower oil

• In a heavy-bottomed skillet gently fry the fillets skin-side down until the skin in golden brown. Remove from the heat and set aside.

• In another pan fry the shallot and red pepper in a little oil until the shallot starts to soften, and then add the garlic purée.

• Cook for a couple of minutes, stirring to prevent the garlic burning, then add the chopped tomato and baby clams.

• Raise the heat and add the wine, allowing the mixture to bubble for a couple of minutes.

• Next, add the stock and dried laver. Stir in thoroughly and allow to heat through.

• Put the skillet containing the fried fish fillet back over a medium heat, and add the sauce ingredients.

• Cover the pan and simmer for a further 10 to 15 minutes. Serve.

JOHN DORY and POTATO-SEAWEED BAKE

2 medium size potatoes
1 small onion
½-1 cup young sugar kelp or dabberlocks
Pepper
1 cup fish / vegetable stock
2 John dory fillets
Unsalted butter / sunflower oil
Dried sea lettuce / laver, finely crushed

If the seaweed is not already sufficiently young and tender you may want to par-boil it for 5 minutes before incorporating with the potato-onion mixture which is then oven cooked like dauphinoise potatoes.

• Begin by peeling and thinly slicing the potatoes.

• Next, thinly slice the onions, and then thinly slice the seaweed.

• Lightly butter or oil a shallow ovenproof dish of a suitable size to hold the sliced potato and onion.

• Next, place a layer of potato on the bottom of the ovenproof dish, followed by a scattered layer of seaweed, then some onions, and lastly a little pepper seasoning. Repeat this layering process until the three ingredients are used up.

• Pour the stock over the potatoes, dot a few small pieces of butter across the top, and then bake in a pre-heated moderately hot (180°C) oven for 50 to 60 minutes, or until the potato is cooked. Once done, remove from the oven, cover with foil, and keep warm.

• Next, melt some butter in a frying pan over a high heat, then shallow fry the fish fillets skin-side down for about 2 to 3 minutes. Turn the fish over with a spatula and cook for another 2 to 3 minutes.

• Serve with the potato-seaweed boulangere, sprinkled with a little dried crushed laver, or sea lettuce sprigs.

SEAWEED RISOTTO

1 small shallot, finely chopped
Garlic purée, to taste
Butter
1 cup Arborio rice
½ cup white wine
½ cup seaweed, shredded
2 cups fish stock, warmed
½ cup peeled prawns
1 small can baby clams, drained

The seaweed here can be mixed, just so long as the fronds are tender. If in doubt, then par-boil the seaweed in water for 5 minutes or as long as the seaweed type dictates. The fish ingredients for this recipe are not hard and fast. Crayfish tails and shrimps could be used, as could squid or octopus suitably prepared and the cooking time amended.

While on the subject of risotto, seaweed may be added to any seafood paella recipe where you want to explore broadening the ingredient base. In this case some of the thicker seaweed species (kelps, sugar kelp, dabberlocks) may be usefully employed as they can take advantage of the longer cooking time to make them tender.

• Begin by frying the shallot in a little butter until it starts to soften, then add the garlic purée and cook for a further minute.

• Stir in the rice and cook for a minute or two then add the wine. Bring to the boil stirring continually.

• Next, add the seaweed and 1 cup of stock. Stir thoroughly and bring to the boil for a couple of minutes.

• Reduce the heat to a simmer, cover the pan, and cook for about 12 to 15 minutes. Add the remaining cup of stock a bit at a time, until it is all absorbed.

• When the rice is tender stir in the cooked prawns and baby clams. Cover the pan and allow to heat through for 2 or 3 minutes, then serve (potentially garnished with sautéd squid or octopus pieces).

MACKEREL, BEAN and SEAWEED RICE

2-4 fresh mackerel fillets
½-1 cup frozen broad beans
Sea lettuce
1 small onion, chopped
½ garlic clove, pasted
Oil
Water
1-2 cups cooked long-grain rice

Other fine, leafy, seaweed fronds can substitute here, but the green of the sea lettuce works nicely with the broad bean coloration. Depending on the size of the fish you may want two or four fillets.

• Begin by grilling the mackerel, until the meat is cooked through. Allow to cool, then flake the flesh and set aside.

• Meanwhile, boil the broad beans until tender. Remove from the water with a slotted spoon and when cool, shuck the skins from the beans. Set aside.

• Cut several sea lettuce fronds into squares no larger than about 1-inch wide, and drop these into the still hot bean cooking water.

• In a heavy-bottomed pan stir-fry the onion until almost softened then add the pasted garlic and cook for a few minutes more, then reduce the heat.

• Using a slotted spoon remove the seaweed from the pan and add to the onion-garlic mixture along with a little of the water. Raise the heat and stir the mixture thoroughly.

• Add the reserved beans and rice. Mix thoroughly.

• Stir in the flaked mackerel and allow the mixture to warm through. Serve.

ACKEE, SEAWEED and FISH

1 can ackee, drained
½ cup sea lettuce or gutweed, shredded
½-1 cup white fish, flaked
Butter or oil
½ spring onion (optional)
¼-½ red chilli pepper (optional)

In the West Indies, particularly Jamaica, ackee with saltfish is a popular dish. In botanical terms the ackee is a 'fruit' growing on a shrub or tree, but is used as a vegetable and has the colour and texture of scrambled egg. Fresh ackee fruits have to be prepared carefully since they contain toxins, but they are available canned from some high street supermarket chains, and also ethnic food shops. Canned ackee tends to be crumbly and fragile so needs to be incorporated with care – unless you don't mind a fine scrambled egg appearance.

In Jamaica salt fish is traditionally used, but for this recipe I have often used those surplus, tapering, scrap ends of filleted cod, pollock, whiting, or other white fish. Nothing goes to waste, right?

• Begin by dropping the shredded seaweed in boiling water for a couple of minutes, then drain and set aside.

• If using the red chilli, lightly fry this in a little oil until it just begins to soften, then remove from the pan and set aside.

• Next, fry the flaked fish until it lightly browns and little bits crispen here and there.

• Return the red chilli to the pan, and also the sliced spring onion if using. Cook for a couple of minutes over a medium heat, or until the spring onion is softened. Then remove the mixture from the pan and keep warm.

• Next, add shredded seaweed to the pan, and crumble and fold in the ackee (break it up with a fork for a finer texture). Cook until the ackee is warmed through. Plate the ackee-seaweed then spoon over the chilli-fish mixture and serve.

A curried version of this may be produced by using 1 small, chopped, shallot as a non-optional ingredient replacement for the spring onion, ½ cup coconut milk, chilli as a non-option, and ½ to 1 teaspoon of curry powder of preferred strength.

SEAWEED FU-YUNG

¼ cup finely shredded seaweed
¼ cup cooked prawns or shrimps, peeled
3 medium eggs
2-3 tsp. light soy sauce
Mirin, dash
Sunflower oil

The type of seaweed used for this recipe needs to be one of the tender species such as sea lettuce, gutweed or young dulse.

• Beat the eggs is a mixing bowl, then fold in the prawns and seaweed.

• Next, add a dash of mirin and the soy sauce, and stir through the egg mixture.

• Heat a little oil in a skillet or wok, and when very hot pour in the egg mixture. Toss and stir-try for 3 or 4 minutes, or until the eggs are cooked through, then serve.

SEAWEED FRIED RICE

1 cup rice, cooked
¼ cup seaweed
¼ cup cooked shrimps, peeled
1 medium egg, beaten
1 tsp. onion, grated
Sunflower oil

A tender and delicate seaweed species should be used here to accompany the shrimps (note, not prawns, just good old seaside shrimps). If opting for a more substantial seaweed species then pre-cook the fronds until just tender and then incorporate as an ingredient. This is really a side dish or starter, but could be turned into a main course by upping the ingredient quantities.

• Begin by cutting or shredding the seaweed into small pieces. Set aside.

• Heat a little oil in a medium-size pan and fry the onion until it is soft, then add the seaweed and shrimps. Stir-fry for a few minutes, then take off the heat and cover to keep warm.

• Heat another small amount of oil in a skillet or wok then stir-fry the rice for a couple of minutes.

• Next, stir the beaten egg into the rice and continue cooking until the egg is cooked through, using a fork to scramble the egg.

• Add the seaweed-shrimp mixture to the pan, turn up the heat, and stir-fry for a few minutes, then serve.

SEA LETTUCE with PRAWNS

4 tiger prawns
½ cup sea lettuce, sliced
¼ cup cucumber, sliced

2-3 tsp. rice vinegar
2-3 tsp. light soy sauce
1 tsp. caster sugar
1 tsp. stem ginger, pasted

A substitute for the sea-lettuce here would be the outer border part of young sugar kelp. Although the prawns are cooked in boiling water in this instance, they could also be grilled or broiled.

• Slice the seaweed into lengths of about 2 or 3 inches, and about the width of a pencil (or tagliatelli thickness), then drop into boiling water. Boil for a couple of minutes, then reduce the heat to a gentle simmer. Cook for another 5 minutes, then drain, refresh with cold water, drain again and set aside.

• Meanwhile, de-vein the prawns (the tails can be left on) and cook in another pan of boiling water until done, using just enough water to cover them. When done, remove from the pan and allow to cool.

• Peel a piece of cucumber about 1½ to 2 inches long, then slice very thinly into rounds and place in a bowl.

• Add the chilled seaweed to the bowl.

• Next, make a dressing with the remaining ingredients, ensuring the sugar is fully dissolved. Drizzle this over the vegetable ingredients in the bowl and toss with a fork.

• Place heaps of the salad vegetables on plates and the prawns on top. Serve.

SEAWEED and YELLOW BEAN FISH BALLS

1 cup white fish fillet, boned
1 medium egg white
3 tsp. cornflour
Pepper
½ spring onion, finely sliced
¼ cup sea lettuce / dabberlocks, finely chopped

2 tsp. yellow bean sauce
½ cup fish stock
1-2 tsp. light soy sauce
Rice wine, splash
1 tsp. sesame oil

If dabberlocks is being used for this recipe then only the most tender, young, outer parts of small fronds should be used not the midrib, while a young sugar kelp frond may substitute too. Minced dace is sometimes available from Chinese supermarkets which saves valuable preparation time.

• Cut the fish into pieces and place in a food processor bowl, along with the egg white, cornflour, and a little pepper seasoning. Blend until a smooth paste forms.

• Add the spring onion and chopped seaweed, and fold into the paste with a fork.

• Form the paste into 1-inch balls, placing each one on a plate and then place them in a refrigerator to chill for 30 minutes.

• Next, bring some water to the boil in a pan, reduce to a simmer and poach the fish balls until they rise to the top, usually about 3 to 4 minutes. Remove with a slotted spoon, allow to drain, and set aside.

• Put the remaining sauce ingredients in a skillet (or wok), bring to the boil, then add the fish balls and stir-fry for a few minutes.

• Serve with rice.

STEAMED FISH, BLACK BEANS and SEAWEED

2 white fish fillets or steaks
2-3 tsp. rice wine vinegar
Sea lettuce leaves (or nori)
Sunflower oil
3-4 tsp. Chinese fermented black beans
1 tsp. stem ginger, thinly sliced
1 small spring onion, thinly sliced
½ garlic clove, pasted
2 tbsp. light soy sauce
1 tbsp. water or fish stock
Chilli / pepper sauce, to taste
Sesame oil (optional)

Coley, pollock and cod may be used for this recipe which uses black fermented beans, not soaked and cooked black beans. The fermented bean version is a quite pungent condiment, and potentially you could replace it with other preserved bean condiments, or try substituting the flavour of black bean sauce from a supermarket shelf – yet another bean condiment flavouring.

The procedure here requires a bit of culinary dexterity since the fish needs to be steamed using basic equipment. Alternatively use a bespoke fish steamer and make up the sauce in a separate pan, spooning the sauce over the fish parcels as they are served.

• Cut the fillets into finger sized lengths and place on a plate.

• Next, drizzle the fish with the rice wine, rub into the flesh and then wrap each piece of fish in a sea lettuce (or nori) frond.

• Select a heatproof plate big enough to fit in your frying pan, while large enough to hold the fish parcels. To support the plate in the pan use a cake trivet, cooling rack or saucepan stand.

• Lightly oil the plate surface then place the fish parcels on the plate.

• Next, pour about an inch of boiling kettle water into the bottom of the frying pan. Carefully lower the plated fish into the pan, bring the water to the boil, then cover and steam the fish for 10 to 15 minutes, or until done (thickness will ultimately determine timing).

• Meanwhile, rinse the black beans and set aside.

• When the fish is done, carefully remove the plate, cover with kitchen foil, and keep the parcels warm.

• Tip out the remaining cooking water, then add a splash of sunflower oil to the pan. Stir-fry the ginger, spring onion, garlic and black beans very briefly.

• Add soy sauce, water and chilli sauce to taste, mix thoroughly and bring to the boil for a minute or so. Add a splash of sesame oil if using.

• Serve with the sauce spooned over the fillets.

SEAWEED and FISH DUMPLINGS

1 cup white fish meat
1 medium egg yolk
3 tsp. cornflour
¼ cup sea lettuce / gutweed, finely chopped
Pepper
1 pint fish stock
Water, boiling
½ spring onion, finely sliced
½ garlic clove, pasted
2-3 tsp. light soy sauce
1 tbsp. dry cooking sherry
2 tsp. sweet chilli sauce
2-3 tsp. sour cream

• Break the fish into pieces, place in a bowl, along with the egg yolk and corn flour, and blend with a food processor until a smooth-ish paste forms (reduce fineness for more texture).

• Stir in the chopped seaweed, and add some seasoning.

• Place the mixture in a refrigerator for 30 minutes then form into 1-inch balls with your hands (keeping your hands moistened with water makes the process less messy too).

• Meanwhile, in a small pan sweat the garlic and spring onion till the onion softens, then add the soy, sherry and chilli sauce, and cook for about a minute more. Remove from the heat.

• Next, bring the fish stock to the boil in a pan (add more boiling water if required) and poach the seaweed-fish dumplings for 4 or 5 minutes. Drain the dumplings with a slotted spoon, cover, and keep warm.

• Return the sauce back to a gentle heat and stir in the sour cream. Serve this sauce spooned over the dumplings.

SEAWEED FISH CAKES

½ cup crab meat, boned
½ cup fresh pollock meat, boned
½-1 tsp. galangal paste
½ garlic clove, minced
¼ cup dulse, finely shredded
1 tsp. chopped red chilli
1 spring onion, sliced thinly
Oil

Galangal is a plant related to ginger but has a more peppery taste, sometimes with a hint of citrus. When living in London I was able to get fresh galangal roots from a Thai supermarket down the road, but these days it is sometimes available fresh from high street supermarkets, and also as a paste. Galangal may also be bought in powder form, and as dried slices. The final outcome of this dish can be quite fierce on the taste-buds – in a pleasant way, of course – so regard the quantity here as allowing you to pace yourself without overdoing galangal as an ingredient.

• If the pollock or crab is moist, dry if off on kitchen paper, cut into pieces and then place these in a food processor bowl along with the galangal paste and minced garlic. Blend till a thick, rough, paste forms (thinner for a smoother texture).

• Next, fold in the dulse, red chilli and spring onion with a fork, making sure these are thoroughly distributed.

• Take about a heaped tablespoon of the mixture and form into patties or fish cakes, place on a lightly oiled baking dish, and cook in a pre-heated moderate oven (180°C) for about 15 to 20 minutes, or until cooked through.

SEAWEED-TOFU PARCELS

1 packet extra firm tofu
¼ cup cooked prawns or shrimps
¼ cup tender seaweed, finely chopped / shredded
Tabasco
Light soy sauce
Sunflower oil
Sesame oil

The idea behind this recipe is for a snack-type finger food, although the parcels could be incorporated into a salad. The amount of seaweed and shellfish may be altered to accommodate tofu pack size, which may vary depending on the brand.

• Carefully cut the firm tofu block in half along its length with a sharp knife. Then halve each along the width. (You should have four pieces about 3 inches square and up to about ¼-inch deep, depending on block thickness. With thicker tofu blocks you may get six pieces).

• Cover a large plate or baking tray with cling film and put the tofu pieces on this, making sure the pieces do not touch. Cover with another sheet of cling film and freeze for several hours, preferably longer.

• Remove the tofu from the freezer and defrost on paper towel, and pat dry to remove excess moisture.

• Meanwhile, finely chop or paste the prawns (or even some other fish) in a bowl with a few drops of Tabasco, and then mix in the shredded seaweed.

• Next, using a sharp pointed knife, carefully cut a pocket into each tofu piece, then brush or rub the pieces with soy sauce.

• Put a little sunflower oil in a frying pan and a spot of sesame oil, and pan-fry the tofu over a medium heat for several minutes on each side.

• Remove from the heat, and when cool enough to handle tease the pockets open and stuff with 1 or 2 teaspoons of the prawn-seaweed mixture.

• Place the stuffed tofu pieces on a lightly oiled baking tray, or non-stick baking sheet, and bake in a pre-heated, moderately-hot oven (190°C) for about 10 minutes or until golden brown.

WHITING / SOLE CEVICHE

2 whiting or sole fillets, skinned
1 small lime, juiced
1-2 tbsp. rice vinegar
Sea lettuce / sugar kelp
½ cup broad beans
½ cup tofu, sliced or cubed
2-3 tsp. light soy sauce
1-2 tsp. walnut oil

Collect, or use, just enough sea lettuce or the outer border area of a very young sugar kelp frond, to cover the fish fillets. Any surplus seaweed could, potentially, be added to the bean-tofu salad, though you might find there is something of a seaweed overkill. If the sugar kelp is slightly tough par-boil it in salted water until tender then refresh in cold water before use in the recipe.

• Place the fillets on a plate.

• Combine the rice vinegar and lime juice (reserving 1-2 tsp.), drizzle over the fish, then turn the fillets over a couple of times to ensure they are coated with the marinade.

• Cover with cling film and place in a refrigerator for 30 minutes. After 30 minutes carefully turn the cooking fillets over, and chill for a further 30 minutes.

• Pod the beans and boil in salted water until tender, then drain, refresh with cold water and shell them. Set aside.

• Meanwhile, wash the seaweed and lay it flat on a work surface.

• Also, slice or cube (small sugar-lump size) the tofu and place in a bowl, along with the shelled beans.

• Remove the fillets from the fridge and drain off the marinade.

• Place a seaweed frond flat on a cutting board and using a spatula lay the first fish fillet on the frond.

• Cover this with a second seaweed frond, then lay the second fillet on top, and finally the third seaweed frond over the top fillet. Trim off surplus seaweed (even square up the fillets if you want to present the dish as a neat sushi).

• Next, with a very sharp knife cut the sandwiched fillets into finger width slices – increasing the width towards the tail ends. Place on the serving plate.

• Make a dressing of the reserved lime juice, soy and walnut oil and drizzle over the bean-tofu salad.

• Serve this alongside the seaweed-fish slices.

More of a salad, but still a ceviche, is a **PRAWN and SEAWEED CEVICHE** in which raw, cleaned, prawns are marinaded for 15 minutes in lemon juice. Meanwhile, soak wakame in water (4 or 5 minutes), then prepare the vegetables: the red onion, cut into thin strips; de-seeded green chilli, thinly sliced; and cucumber, peeled, de-seeded and sliced into semi-circles. Place these in a bowl, add the drained wakame, marinaded prawns and lemon juice, toss with a fork and serve.

SOBA NOODLES with CRISPY SEAWEED

Soba (Buckwheat) noodles
1 salmon fillet
2 tbsp. light soy sauce
2 tbsp. mirin
2 tbsp. dry sherry
2-3 tsp. ginger root, pasted
½-1 cup gutweed
Sunflower oil
Sesame oil

Buckwheat noodles are darker than other noodles – such as egg and udon – traditionally used in Asian cooking, while gutweed has an uncanny knack of harbouring the finest sandy particles and needs to be thoroughly washed several times. Before frying the seaweed it should be patted dry on kitchen paper otherwise it may spit violently when put into hot oil.

Some further ways of frying seaweeds will be found on page 81 and might provide you with alternative ideas to serve with this recipe.

• Cook enough noodles for 2 helpings according to packet instructions. When done, drain, refresh with cold water, drain again, and set aside.

• Cut the salmon fillet into very thin slices (think of smoked salmon thickness) and layer the pieces in a shallow dish.

• Next, make a marinade in a small dish with the sherry, soy sauce, mirin and pasted ginger. Mix the ingredients thoroughly and pour over the salmon slices, gently turning the pieces so the liquid reaches both sides of the slices. Then cover with cling film and allow to marinate for 30 minutes.

• Then tease the gutweed fronds apart – as they may be compressed from drying on kitchen paper – and deep fry in hot oil for about 10 to 20 seconds (test cook a few fronds before doing the whole volume). Remove from the pan with a slotted spoon and place on kitchen paper to drain.

• Next, drain the marinade off the salmon slices, but reserve the liquid.

• Put a little sesame and sunflower oil in the bottom of a non-stick frying pan, heat and swirl around, then layer the salmon slices in the bottom of the pan. Allow to cook through without turning. Then use a suitable non-scratch fish slice to remove the cooked salmon pieces. Set aside and keep warm.

• Next, add a good slug of sunflower oil to the pan, raise the heat, then add the noodles and reserved marinade and stir-fry for several minutes until the noodles are heated through.

• Serve the noodles heaped on a plate, with the fried gutweed placed on top and the salmon pieces dotted around.

CELLOPHANE NOODLES and SEAWEED

Cellophane noodles, cooked
½ cup seaweed – sea lettuce, sugar kelp
½-1 cup cooked prawns, shrimps
1 tsp. grated ginger root
2 tbsp. rice vinegar
1 tbsp. light soy sauce
1 tsp. sugar

Dried vermicelli rice noodles could be used as an alternative here, and need practically no cooking – other than the boiling water they are soaked in. Although cellophane noodles look somewhat pale, like rice noodles, they are made from mung bean starch and do need cooking. Where sugar kelp is used then this will need some pre-cooking before inclusion as an ingredient.

• Prepare enough of the noodles for two portions according to pack instructions, then drain, run under cold water, drain again and place in a mixing bowl. Using kitchen scissors cut the noodles into 2 to 3-inch lengths.

• Next, chop the seaweed then add to the noodles.

• Add the prawns or shrimps to the bowl and distribute the ingredients thoroughly with a fork.

• In a small dish mix the grated ginger, vinegar, soy sauce and sugar. Drizzle over the noodle mixture, gently toss to coat the noodles with the dressing then serve.

SEAWEED PILAU

½ cup seaweed
1 cup basmati rice
Saffron, small pinch
1 small shallot, finely sliced
½ tsp. red chilli, finely chopped
½ tsp. ginger root, grated
Sunflower oil
½-1 cups shrimps or prawns, cooked
Cinnamon bark
2 bay leaves
2 green cardamom pods

Depending on whether you are using one of the tender seaweed varieties or more robust ones the cooking method will differ. Add the tender ones to the rice in the last stage of the recipe, while the tougher ones should be cooked along with the basmati rice at the start. Really robust seaweeds should be pre-cooked before use.

• Slice, chop or shred the seaweed into whatever visual shape you prefer. Set aside.

• Next, boil the rice in water (add tougher seaweeds at this stage) and when the rice is about half-cooked take off the heat, drain – but reserve the cooking water – and set aside.

• Take ½ cup of the reserved water and add a pinch of saffron threads to soak.

• Meanwhile, cut the shallot lengthways then fry in a heavy-bottomed skillet until the pieces begin to soften, then add the chilli and ginger. Continue stir-frying until the shallot starts to turn golden brown.

• Add the prawns or shrimps and stir fry for a 2 or 3 minutes.

• Add the half-cooked rice to the pan and stir thoroughly (add more tender seaweeds at this point), plus a piece of cinnamon bark, bay leaves, and the saffron water.

• Stir the mixture well, then cover the pan and cook over a medium-low heat until the rice is tender, then serve.

SEAWEED and FISH CURRY

½ cup sea spaghetti (thongweed), young shoots
1 small shallot, thinly sliced
Sunflower oil
2-3 tsp. mild curry paste
½ cup chicken stock
1 cup coconut milk
1-2 cups firm white fish, fork-size pieces
1 spring onion, sliced

• Boil the sea spaghetti shoots for 10 minutes, then remove from the heat, drain, and set aside.

• Stir-fry the shallot in a little oil until soft, then mix in the curry paste, the chicken stock and sea spaghetti. Cook for a minute or two.

• Next, add the coconut milk. Stir to ensure even distribution, bring to the boil for a minute, then reduce to a simmer.

• Layer the fish pieces on top of the cooking mixture, and then the spring onion on top of this.

• Cover the frying pan, and cook at a medium heat for 10 to 12 minutes, or until the fish is cooked through.

• Then gently fold the fish into the seaweed-curry sauce with a fork, and serve with rice.

SEAWEED, FISH and COCONUT CURRY

½ cup sea spaghetti (thongweed), young shoots
1 small shallot, minced
1 small green pepper
Sunflower oil
1-2 tsp. mild curry powder / paste
1-2 tsp. stem ginger, pasted
Green Tabasco sauce (optional)
1 cup coconut milk
1½-2 cups firm white fish meat, fork-size

A firm white fish such as cod or monkfish is called for here, and should be cut into fork-size chunks. Red and yellow pepper may also be used, but since the seaweed here is a green species then green pepper is in colour harmony. Where grated root ginger is used as a substitute, add a few small pinches of sugar to the cooking coconut milk. Towards the end of cooking you may add a little hot water where you prefer a more gravy-like sauce consistence.

• Cut the sea spaghetti into 1½ to 2-inch pieces, then drop into boiling water. Cook for a minute, then reduce to a simmer.

• Meanwhile, briskly stir-fry the shallot and pepper in a little oil.

• Stir in the curry paste, ginger, and a little Tabasco (adds a little extra, but mild, heat), and cook for another minute. Then take off the heat while you deal with the seaweed.

• Check the sea spaghetti is cooked, but still has a 'bite' to it. Drain the seaweed.

• Return the shallot and spices mixture to the heat, and stir in the drained seaweed pieces.

• Stir in the coconut milk, bring the mixture to the boil for minute, then reduce to a simmer.

• Add the fish pieces to the pan, cover, and cook for another 10 to 15 minutes or until the fish is cooked through. Serve with rice.

SPICED FISH with KELP

2 white fish fillets
½-1 cup seaweed – sugar kelp, dabberlocks
2-3 tbsp. rice vinegar
Caster sugar, pinch
1-3 tbsp. sultanas
¼-½ tsp. red chilli, finely sliced
½ tsp. ginger root, pasted
Garlic purée, to taste (optional)

• Cut the fish into good fork-size pieces, and set aside.

• Add a spot of hot water to the sultanas, in a small dish, to puff them up.

• Cut the seaweed into manageable size pieces, then drop into boiling water and cook till tender. The remove with a slotted spoon, refresh in cold water, drain, and set aside.

• Next, cook the fish pieces in the same water for about 3 or 4 minutes, or until done. Then remove the fish with a slotted spoon and set aside.

• Make a dressing with the rice vinegar, sugar, sultanas, ginger, sliced chilli, and garlic (if using) and mix everything together well.

• To serve the dish, heap the seaweed on a plate, place the fish pieces on top of this, and then spoon the dressing over.

PRAWN and SEAWEED CURRY

1 small red shallot, minced
Garlic purée, to taste (optional)
1 tsp. grated ginger root
1 tbsp. Thai red curry paste
Sunflower oil
1 cup coconut milk
Fish sauce
¼ cup dulse, sliced
1 cup cooked prawns / crayfish, peeled

This recipe plays with the visual appearance of the red and pink colours of the ingredients. Smaller shrimps can be used in substitution for the prawns and crayfish.

• Lightly stir-fry the shallot in a little oil for a couple of minutes, then add the garlic (if using) and ginger. Cook for another couple of minutes, making sure to stir the mixture.

• Next, add the curry paste and continue cooking for a couple of minutes.

• Stir in the coconut milk, dulse, and a small splash of fish sauce. Bring to the mixture briefly to the boil, then reduce the heat to a simmer.

• Add the cooked prawns and crayfish, stir well, and cover the pan. Cook for several more minutes to ensure the shellfish are warmed through. Serve with rice.

SEAWEED and OCTOPUS MACARONI

Macaroni, or penne
½-1 cup seaweed
1 small can octopus or baby squid
½ shallot, sliced
Garlic, pasted
½ tsp. red chilli, finely sliced
Oil
½ cup white wine
1 tbsp. tomato purée
Warm water
Pepper

For this recipe the seaweed should be one of the tender types which require little cooking. If opting for more robust species (such as the kelps) then these should be pre-cooked until just tender, then reserved for use at the appropriate later point in the recipe.

• When using robust seaweeds then start pre-cooking them by boiling in water at the beginning. Test from time to time (they want to be slightly underdone), drain and set aside at the appropriate tenderness.

• Meanwhile, cook enough pasta for 2 servings according to pack instructions and almost at the al dente point (very slightly underdone). Set aside.

• Check through the contents of the tinned octopus / squid, cutting any large pieces into smaller fork-size pieces.

• Slice half a shallot lengthways, then fry in a little oil (which may come from the tinned fish) in a medium-size frying pan until golden brown.

• Next, add the chilli and garlic to the pan and stir-fry for a minute.

• Then add the white wine and allow the mixture to come to the boil.

• Dilute the tomato purée in about 1 cup of warm water and stir into the pan's contents. Allow everything to come to the boil.

• Add the cooked pasta and seaweed to the pan, stir in thoroughly, and season with pepper.

• Cook for about 5 minutes, then add the drained octopus / squid and fold through the mixture.

• Continue cooking for a further 5 minutes then serve.

MACKEREL, MACARONI and SEAWEED FRITTATA

1 smoked mackerel fillet
¼ cup young sugar kelp, finely chopped
½ cup frozen peas
1-2 cups cooked macaroni
2 or 3 medium eggs
Milk
Oil
Pepper

• Drop the sugar kelp into a small pan of boiling water and cook for about 5 minutes (increase time accordingly when not using the youngest frond material).

• Meanwhile, skin and bone the mackerel fillet, then flake the meat. Set aside.

• Take the cooked kelp off the heat and remove the seaweed with a slotted spoon. Drain, and set aside.

• Next, cook the peas in the same water for a few minutes, then remove from the heat, drain, and set aside to cool.

• In a mixing bowl, whisk the eggs with a little milk and season with pepper.

• Add the seaweed and peas to the bowl, and fold in with a fork.

• Fold in the flaked mackerel, and then the cooked macaroni, and make sure all the ingredients are thoroughly distributed.

• Next, place some oil in a frying pan and when hot turn out the seaweed-pasta mixture, levelling the ingredients evenly in the bottom of the pan.

• Cook over a medium heat until the bottom is golden brown then, using a plate, flip the frittata over and cook the other side for several minutes, then serve.

While on the topic of pasta, I wonder whether the **SEAWEED PESTO** on page 78 might make some sort of interesting filling for handmade ravioli; small amounts mixed with a fish ingredient, or perhaps traces with minced beef for a filling.

SEAWEED VONGOLE

1 small shallot
Garlic purée, to taste
Olive oil
1 tbsp. seaweed, finely chopped
½ cup fish stock
1 can small baby clams, drained
Dry white wine
Pepper
Spaghetti

Young dulse, dabberlocks, sugar kelp, or virtually any other tender sea-weed may be used here, including young sprouts of sea spaghetti. Where using the latter as an ingredient, cut it into 2-inch lengths to mimic the form of the real pasta.

• Lightly fry the shallot until soft, then add the garlic and cook for a further minute or two, stirring to prevent burning.

• Add the chopped seaweed and fish stock, and briefly bring to the boil.

• Reduce the heat and simmer for 5 to 10 minutes.

• Meanwhile, start cooking the spaghetti (2 portions) according to pack instructions, until al dente.

• Next, add the baby clams to the frying pan, a good slug of white wine, and a little pepper seasoning. Simmer gently for a few minutes, until the clams are warmed through.

• Drain the cooked pasta and add to the clam-seaweed sauce.

• Mix everything thoroughly, and serve – dusting with a little seaweed salt / sea spice if fancied.

Sea Spice is nothing really more than dried seaweed ground down to the consistency of salt. As long as the seaweed is bone dry it is quite easy to make at home in a coffee grinder, or similar. It is a good way of using up scraps of dried seaweed lurking in your kitchen cupboard.

SEAWEED-PASTA BAKE

Spaghetti pasta
1 cup cooked fish meat, finely flaked
½-1 cup seaweed, shredded / chopped
Black olives, sliced (optional)
Pepper
Cream
1 cup white breadcrumbs
Olive oil

The idea for this recipe originated with a Spanish way of using pasta *fideos* – finger length pieces of spaghetti-type pasta. For simplicity, use an ordinary fine gauge spaghetti and break it into 2 to 3-inch lengths for this recipe. I tried this with wholegrain pasta but it doesn't really work as it makes the dish rather 'heavy going', well in my view. As with many recipes in this book various seaweed species may be used here as the sea vegetable ingredient, but the more substantial ones will need some pre-cooking.

• Begin by cooking enough pasta for two servings, according to pack instructions, until just al dente. Then drain and set aside.

• Flake the fish in a bowl with a fork (the consistency I look for is where individual flakes become broken into a really fibrous texture, but not a purée-like consistency).

• Add the seaweed to the bowl, and a few sliced black olives if using, and the cooked pasta. Mix everything thoroughly with a fork.

• Oil or butter a shallow, suitably sized, ovenproof dish, then fill with the pasta-fish mixture.

• Add a little pepper seasoning, then drizzle over about 1 or 2 tablespoons of cream.

• Sprinkle the breadcrumbs over the pasta and drizzle over a little olive oil.

• Bake in a pre-heated moderate oven (180°C) for 25 to 30 minutes, then serve.

SEAWEED and ANCHOVY BUTTER

¼ cup unsalted butter
2 or 3 anchovy fillets
2-3 tbsp. dulse, finely chopped
Cayenne, pinch

This butter may either be spread on toasted bread, added to a sauce in a fish recipe, or knobs of the mixture served on top of plated fish fillets or cutlets. To really allow the seaweed flavour to permeate the mixture it should be prepared several hours ahead of use. Overnight would be even better.

• Begin by creaming the butter in a small bowl.

• Next, cut the anchovy fillets small and place in a pestle and mortar, and pound them.

• Add the fish to the creamed butter, followed by the chopped dulse and cayenne. Mix thoroughly with a fork.

• Cover in cling film and chill in the refrigerator before use.

AGAR AGAR SEAWEED MEDLEY

Crab meat
Seaweed, blanched and finely chopped
Carrot, blanched and finely chopped
Agar agar
Rice vinegar
Soy sauce
Mirin

This recipe uses *agar agar* and is left intentionally open-ended since agar can appear in different strengths so you will need to follow specific pack instructions on volumes and measurements.

• The 'concept', however, is to set the seaweed, carrot and fish ingredients in agar jelly, very much as would happen with aspic or gelatine.

• Once set the jelly is cubed as a salad or snack item, with a flavourful dressing created from the rice vinegar, soy sauce and mirin.

While agar agar is not a physical seaweed it is made from seaweed, and has properties similar to Irish Moss or Carragheen (*Chondrus crispus*) as a gelling agent. The inclusion of agar in this book is simply because this ingredient allows for the creation of other types of dishes and, in my view, is infinitely easier to prepare when compared to the rigmarole involved in extracting the gelling properties of Irish Moss.

When reconstituted agar is almost a clear, colourless, gel, and has no taste or smell. Unlike gelatine the texture of agar is more firm, rougher textured, and remains as a jelly up to temperatures of around 80°C.

So, agar agar is another vegetable equivalent of gelatin but made from seaweed, and for that reason is useful in vegetarian diets. Generally available in powder and flaked forms from supermarkets, some health food shops, and Asian stores, agar finds uses in everything from making fruit preserves, to desserts, ice cream, as a thickener for soups, as an emulsifier and stabilizer in the food industry, and sometimes in cakes and breads where the moisture-holding properties of agar may prolong the life of the product. In Asia agar is known as *kanten* (Japan) and China Grass (India), and is often sold in bar or block form, and even in strands like vermicelli noodles. If you decide to hunt down agar then other alternative names to be aware of are Faluda, Japanese or Ceylon Moss, and Bengal Isinglass.

Some pointers on your use of agar / kanten...

Depending on the agar grade, a very rough guide is that 1 tablespoon of agar will thicken 1 cup of a neutral liquid such as milk, water, or stock. Acid liquids, such as fruit juices, will need the quantity of agar increasing, while increases in the amount of dissolved agar produces a more firm, chewy, end result with a higher melting point than gelatine-based items.

Agar is not added to foods directly. Instead, the powder is added to your chosen flavoured liquid, whisked to disperse the granules or powder, brought to the boil then simmered for several minutes – longer in the case of thicker agar flakes. While the agar substrate is still liquid the solid ingredients are added, mixed in, then poured into a suitable mould or moulds, and allowed to set (somewhere around 40°C).

MEAT

BEEF and SEAWEED BROTH

½ cup seaweed, sliced
1 cup beef, shredded wafer thin or ground
½ tsp. garlic, crushed
1 dsp. soy sauce
Sesame oil
Pepper
Sunflower oil
3 or 4 cups water

Two seaweed species are good for this – sea lettuce and very young dulse – though they have different food, stroke cooking, qualities. If using dulse the cooking time needs to be extended since it is a tougher product of the sea than the more fragile sea lettuce. Dabberlocks and young sugar kelp could also come into the ingredient frame here. In my view the latter two need pre-cooking until almost tender then combining with the meat components near the end of the cooking procedure.

• Begin by washing the seaweed, and cutting it into small, teaspoon-size, pieces.

• Next, shred the beef very finely (or even use it in minced / ground form) and place in a bowl with the garlic, soy, a dash of sesame oil and a little pepper.

• Thoroughly incorporate the ingredients then sauté them in a little sun-flower oil until the meat is cooked through.

• Add the seaweed pieces and water, bring to the boil briefly, then reduce to a medium heat and cook for a 5 to 10 minutes, or until the seaweed is tender.

• Finally, amend the seasoning with more pepper and soy as required, and serve.

An alternative to presenting this as a broth is to cut down on the water content and serve it almost as a tapas-like dish.

SEAWEED with MINCED BEEF

½-1 cup dabberlocks, shredded
Vinegar, splash
½ small shallot, finely chopped
Garlic purée, to taste
Ground cumin, pinch
Pepper
Sunflower oil
1 cup minced beef
1 tomato, skinned, chopped
2 tsp. plain flour

Where wakame or another seaweed is used instead of dabberlocks then amend the cooking time to cater for the difference in tenderness.

Incidentally, a friend of mine added pieces of dried wakame to chilli con carne sauce, the liquid re-hydrating the seaweed. By all accounts it made a very good addition and increased the depth of flavour positively. So that is another seaweed-beef combination for you to try.

• Place the seaweed in a small pan with just enough water to submerge it, and add a splash of vinegar.

• Bring to the boil for a minute, then reduce the heat and simmer for 10 minutes. Then drain and set aside.

• Meanwhile, fry the onion over a medium heat until it begins to soften, then add the garlic (to taste) and cumin, and season with a little pepper. Cook for a further 2 or 3 minutes.

• Add the minced beef and stir-fry for several minutes, then add the chopped tomato.

• Continue stir-frying for several minutes then turn the heat down low, cover, and cook for about 15 minutes.

• Raise the heat back to medium, sprinkle the flour over the contents of the pan, distribute thoroughly, and cook until the mixture thickens.

• Lastly, add the drained seaweed, mix in and cook until warmed through.

• Serve with one of the non-fish seaweed salads in this book, or even the Mushroom, Seaweed and Bulgur patties on page 72.

LAVER and CHICKEN BURGERS

2 skinless chicken breasts, minced
½ cup fresh white breadcrumbs
¼ cup dried laver, finely crumbled
1-2 tbsp. minced red onion
1 tbsp. lemon juice
Cayenne, pinch
Sunflower oil

These burgers may be served with a salad, or in buns à la barbeque, and either grilled or pan-fried. Alternatives to cayenne would be the milder sweet paprika, or finely chopped fresh chilli for a nice clean spicy heat.

The laver here will never be properly cooked through, rather it is being used to add its flavour to the background. In this respect, dried dulse would be another alternative seaweed since it is perfectly edible raw in its dried form.

• Place the minced chicken in a mixing bowl, then add all the other ingredients, plus a little cayenne seasoning.

• Mix thoroughly, without the mixture becoming a mush.

• Cover the bowl, and allow to stand for 10 to 15 minutes (allows for a little hydration of the laver).

• Next, form the meat into four equal portions and form into patties.

• Depending on the cooking method, either lightly oil both sides of the patties and then cook under a medium, pre-heated, grill for 5 to 7 minutes per side, or fry in a little oil for about 5 minutes on each side. In either case, the burgers should be cooked until the juices run clear and the meat is no longer pink inside.

PORK TENDERLOIN and GUTWEED

Pork tenderloin
Garlic, crushed, to taste
Salt
½ cup gutweed (or sea lettuce)
1 spring onion, sliced
2-3 tsp. light soy sauce
2-3 tsp. mirin
1-2 tsp. lime juice (optional)

Make sure to give the gutweed several washes as there is a tendency for fine sand to remain lodged in its wrinkled crevices. If using sea lettuce as an alternative, slice it into pencil thickness pieces. Although untried at this moment in time, wakame might be worth trying here.

• Rub the tenderloin (sufficient for 2 servings) with garlic and salt then fry or roast the tenderloin until cooked through. Cover in tinfoil and keep warm.

• Meanwhile, wash the gutweed thoroughly, then drop into boiling water and cook for 5 minutes. Then remove from the heat, drain, and refresh in cold water, and drain again. If the collected seaweed pieces are long then cut into 2 to 3-inch lengths. Set aside.

• Next, cut the paler part of the spring onion into 2 to 3-inch lengths, then quarter lengthways and set aside.

• In a small dish mix the soy, mirin, and lime juice if using. Set aside.

• Uncover the tenderloin and drain the cooking juices into a small sauce boat. Stir in the soy-mirin mixture.

• Slice the tenderloin into medallions and place on the serving plates. Place portions of seaweed and spring onions beside the meat and serve with the gravy-dressing mixture in a sauce dish.

SEAWEED KEBABS

½ small shallot, minced
1 cup cooked prawns
½ cup pork meat
Pepper
Sea lettuce, whole fronds
Sunflower oil
Fish sauce
2 tsp. lime juice
Garlic purée (optional)
Tabasco sauce
Caster sugar, pinch
Bamboo skewers

This recipe calls for sea lettuce to be used as an ingredient wrapping, very much like vine leaves for Greek dolmades, so the sea lettuce leaves need to be sufficiently large enough to wrap the meat ingredients. Where sea lettuce is not available then use the outer border area of a young-ish sugar kelp frond of suitable size, or resort to shop-bought, paper-thin, Japanese nori. Soak the bamboo skewers in water for about 30 minutes to prevent them from scorching, or use metal ones instead.

• Stir-fry the shallot in a small pan until soft, then set aside.

• Next, finely mince the prawns and pork then place in a bowl with a little pepper seasoning.

• Add the cooked shallot to the bowl and a small dash of fish sauce. Mix everything thoroughly.

• Spread individual sea lettuce leaves on the worktop, lightly oil each side facing you, then place a spoonful of the meat mixture on top.

• Wrap the seaweed around as if making dolmades – in all likelihood you will end up with a rag-tag of parcel sizes since sea lettuce from the wilds does not always come in neat, convenient, sizes.

• Fix each parcel on an individual skewer, lightly oil the outer seaweed surface, and cook gently under a pre-heated grill for about 10 to 15 minutes, regularly rotating the kebabs. Keep the heat at a level which does not burn or scorch the seaweed – which tastes dreadful.

• Meanwhile, make up a dipping sauce with about 1 tbsp. of fish sauce, the lime juice, a touch of garlic, a few drops of Tabasco (use the green type for less heat), and a pinch of caster sugar. Serve this alongside the cooked kebabs.

BREADS

SEAWEED CORNBREAD

½ cup cooked sweetcorn kernels
2 cups fine polenta
⅓ cup dried dulse, finely chopped
1 cup whole milk
1 small shallot, finely chopped
5 medium eggs, separated
Butter / sunflower oil
Salt

As an alternative to the lightness provided by the beaten egg whites in this recipe, a tablespoon of baking powder may be used instead. Although not tried, crumbled dried laver might also be a possible altern- ative to the dulse though I particularly like the savoury aspect of dulse as a seaweed ingredient.

• Place the sweetcorn, polenta and dried dulse in a mixing bowl and briefly mix.

• Butter or lightly oil a baking tin or mould.

• Next, fry the shallot in a little oil until softened. Set aside, and when cool add to the sweetcorn-polenta ingredients.

• Meanwhile, beat the egg yolks till well mixed, then whisk the egg whites in another bowl until stiff. Set aside.

• Add the fried onion to the polenta mixture, then pour in the milk and add a pinch of salt. Mix well with a fork.

• Next, stir in the beaten egg yolks, and then fold in the whisked egg whites and distribute thoroughly.

• Pour the mixture into the greased mould and bake at 180°C for about 25 to 30 minutes (a metal skewer inserted into the bread should be clean when removed).

While on the subject of cornbread and sweet corn, add a little chopped dulse to the batter when making sweet corn fritters to accompany Chicken Maryland.

SEAWEED NAAN BREAD

½ tsp. caster sugar
½ tsp. dried yeast
½ cup warm water
¾ cup plain flour
1 tsp. sunflower oil
½ cup dried dulse, finely chopped
Dried laver, powdered or crushed

For a more authentic Indian touch use clarified butter (ghee) instead of the oil.

• Mix the sugar in the warm water and then stir in the yeast. Allow the mixture to stand for 5 to 10 minutes, or until it is frothy.

• Place the flour in a large mixing bowl and add the oil, yeast mixture, and dried dulse. Mix well then knead the mixture into a dough.

• Cover the bowl with cling film and allow the dough to rise for 1 hour in a warm place, or the dough doubles in volume.

• Divide the dough equally into 2 or 4 portions, form into balls, and then roll out on a floured surface till about ¼-inch thick and about 5 or 6 inches wide.

• Brush the top surface of each round with a little oil then place on a lightly oiled baking tray and bake in pre-heated, moderately-hot, oven (200°C) for 10 to 12 minutes.

• Serve with some finely crushed dried laver sprinkled over the bread, or sprinkle with 'sea spice'.

Sea Spice is nothing really more than dried seaweed ground down to the consistency of salt. As long as the seaweed is bone dry it is quite easy to make at home in a coffee grinder, or similar. It is a good way of using up scraps of dried seaweed lurking in your kitchen cupboard.

CHICKPEA-SEAWEED BREADS

½ cup gram / besan / garbanzo (chickpea) flour
½ cup wholemeal flour
Salt, pinch
1 small shallot, minced
¼ cup seaweed, chopped
½ cup water
Sunflower oil, or clarified, unsalted, butter (ghee)

For this recipe use the most tender seaweed species which need little cooking, or try with dried dulse – in which case you may wish to drop the additional salt.

• Sift and mix the two flours in a bowl.

• In a separate dish mix the minced onion and seaweed then add this to the flour, using a fork to distribute through the mixture evenly.

• Add water to the mixture, mix until a dough forms, then cover and set aside for 20 minutes.

• Then kneed the dough for 10 minutes and divide equally into 4 portions.

• Roll the dough into 6-inch patties on a floured board, then lightly oil or butter a frying pan and cook the patties over a medium heat; turning over several times and brushing with a little more oil or butter each time the bread is turned.

SEAWEED BREAD

With regard to 'normal' bread which you may bake at home – or make in a bread-making machine – seaweed makes an excellent savoury addition, and may be added to many of your normal recipes with little need for any changes. Dried dulse is perhaps the best; providing flavour and colour.

The main concern would be using seaweed which is wet, since this alters the moisture content of the dough, while dried seaweed absorbs moisture from the dough. In my view the best option is partly dried wet seaweed, or partly rehydrated. As for quantity, in my view 2 to 4 tablespoons to a small loaf is about right. Your best option is to experiment, starting with one tablespoon added to your first loaf and then increasing the amount each baking day until you reach your preferred quantity.

RECIPE INDEX

FOR YOUR NOTES

www.ingramcontent.com/pod-product-compliance
Lightning Source LLC
Chambersburg PA
CBHW060357290526
45791CB00002B/548